Real English *for* Nurses

기본편

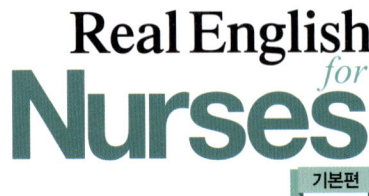

Real English for Nurses 기본편

지은이 Michael A. Putlack, 김진숙, 다락원 ESP 연구소
펴낸이 정규도
펴낸곳 (주)다락원

초판 1쇄 발행 2016년 4월 20일
초판 7쇄 발행 2025년 1월 24일

편집 김태연, 조상익
감수 김희순(서울여자간호대 교수·국제교류센터장)
디자인 장미연, 정규옥

다락원 경기도 파주시 문발로 211
내용문의 (02) 736-2031 내선 550
구입문의 (02) 736-2031 내선 250~252
Fax (02) 732-2037
출판등록 1977년 9월 16일 제406-2008-000007호

Copyright © 2016 Michael A. Putlack

저자 및 출판사의 허락 없이 이 책의 일부 또는 전부를 무단 복제·전재·발췌할 수 없습니다. 구입 후 철회는 회사 내규에 부합하는 경우에 가능하므로 구입문의처에 문의하시기 바랍니다. 분실·파손 등에 따른 소비자 피해에 대해서는 공정거래위원회에서 고시한 소비자 분쟁 해결 기준에 따라 보상 가능합니다. 잘못된 책은 바꿔 드립니다.

ISBN 978-89-277-0909-1 18740
978-89-277-0906-0 18740 (set)

http://www.darakwon.co.kr
다락원 홈페이지를 방문하시면 상세한 출판 정보와 함께 MP3 자료 등의 다양한 어학 정보를 얻으실 수 있습니다.

Real English for Nurses

기본편

Michael A. Putlack, 김진숙,
다락원 ESP 연구소 저

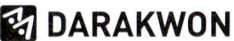

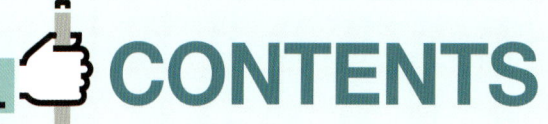

CONTENTS

To the Students

Study Guide

Plan of the Book

UNIT 01	Taking Reservations on the Phone	11
UNIT 02	Receiving Patients	19
UNIT 03	Checking the Conditions of Patients	27
UNIT 04	Giving Directions in and out of Buildings	35
UNIT 05	Examinations I	43
UNIT 06	Examinations II	51
UNIT 07	Giving Orientation about Hospitalization	59
UNIT 08	Taking Care of Patients	67
UNIT 09	Discussing Medication	75
UNIT 10	Reassuring Patients and Guardians	83
UNIT 11	Discharging Patients	91
UNIT 12	Handling Calls from Discharged Patients	99

Answer Key   108

Appendix: Word List   124

To the Students

최근 의료업계는 점점 더 성장하고 있습니다. 이에 따라 간호사라는 직업도 함께 성장하고 있습니다. 요즈음 간호사로서 병원에 취업하고자 하는 이들은 최대한 경쟁력을 높여야 합니다. 이제 단순히 간호 서비스를 제공하는 것만으로는 불충분합니다. 간호사에게도 영어 말하기 능력이 필요한 시대가 되었습니다. 국내 의료 시설에 방문하는 외국인이 점차 늘고 있으며, 외국인 환자에게 최상의 간호 서비스를 제공하기 위해서는 영어로도 의사소통할 수 있어야 하기 때문입니다.

Real English for Nurses 기본편은 병원 취업에 필수적인 영어 표현을 학습할 수 있도록 구성되어 있습니다. 본 교재의 각 유닛은 진료 예약하기, 증상 묻기, 검사하기와 같은 상황을 비롯하여 다양한 주제를 다루고 있습니다. 또한 간호사에게 필요한 핵심 단어 및 표현들도 제공하고 있습니다.

Real English for Nurses 기본편은 일차적으로는 대학 수업용 교재로 개발되었지만, 독학도 가능하도록 구성되어 있습니다. 본 교재는 말하기와 듣기에 중점을 두고 있으며, 독해 및 기초 문법을 다루는 코너도 수록하고 있습니다. Real English for Nurses 기본편으로 꾸준히 학습한다면, 자신도 모르는 사이에 상황에 따라 다양한 영어 표현을 구사할 수 있게 될 것입니다.

Real English for Nurses 기본편을 통해, 영어 실력도 쌓고 병원 취업의 꿈도 이루시기를 진심으로 기원합니다.

다락원 ESP 연구소

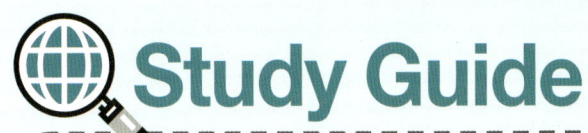

Study Guide

각 유닛은 주제와 관련된 워밍업 활동으로 시작되며, 두 개의 대화문을 중심으로 중요한 단어, 표현, 문법 사항을 학습할 수 있도록 구성되어 있습니다. 뿐만 아니라, 말하기와 듣기 학습을 할 수 있는 활동도 마련되어 있습니다. 마지막으로, 해당 주제와 관련된 독해 지문을 읽어봄으로써 유닛을 마무리할 수 있습니다.

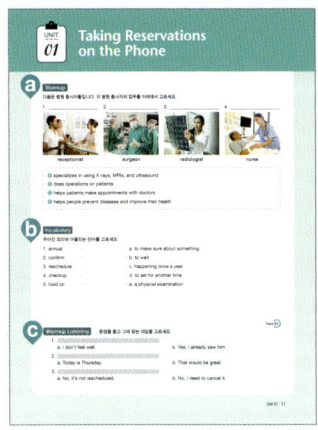
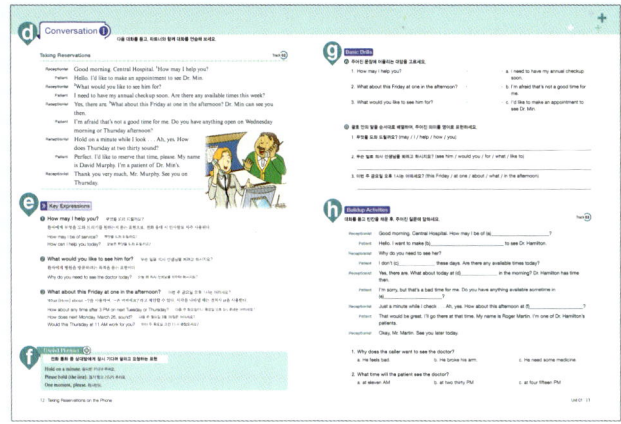

ⓐ Warmup
주제와 관련된 쉽고 흥미로운 활동을 통해 학습을 준비합니다.

ⓑ Vocabulary
대화문의 핵심 단어를 미리 학습해 봅니다.

ⓒ Warmup Listening
대화문의 기본 표현을 미리 학습해 봅니다.

ⓓ Conversation I, II
대화문을 파트너와 함께 연습해 봅니다.

ⓔ Key Expressions
대화문의 핵심 표현 세 가지를 집중적으로 학습합니다.

ⓕ Useful Phrases
대화문과 관련된 추가적인 표현을 학습합니다.

ⓖ Basic Drills
간단한 활동을 통해 배운 내용을 확인합니다.

ⓗ Buildup Activities
받아쓰기 및 문제 풀기를 통해, 앞서 배운 내용을 확실하게 이해합니다.

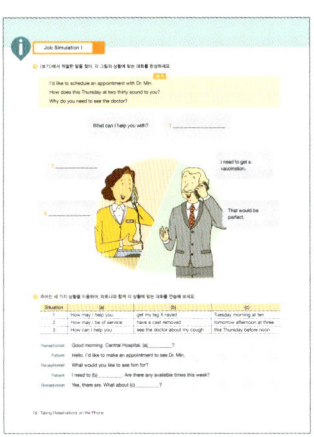
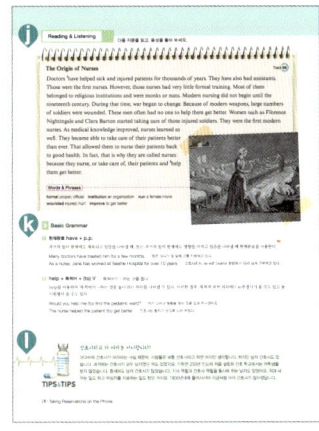

ⓘ Job Simulation I, II
핵심 표현을 응용하여, 배운 내용을 상황에 맞게 적용해 봅니다.

ⓙ Reading & Listening
읽기 및 듣기를 통해, 주제와 관련된 배경지식을 쌓습니다.

ⓚ Basic Grammar
지문의 기본 문법 사항을 학습합니다.

ⓛ TIPS & TIPS
한글로 제공되는 흥미로운 토막글을 통해 해당 분야에 관한 상식을 넓힐 수 있습니다.

Plan of the Book

Unit	Topic	Situations	Language Focus
01	Taking Reservations on the Phone	1. Taking Reservations 2. Changing Reservations	- greeting patients on the telephone - setting up appointments - discussing times and days - making suggestions with "what about" - changing appointments
02	Receiving Patients	1. Receiving Patients 2. Asking Patients about Their Conditions	- greeting patients in person - handling new patients - making suggestions with "why don't you" - asking about symptoms - finding out how long patients have had symptoms
03	Checking the Conditions of Patients	1. Checking Patients' Conditions 2. Checking on Pain	- explaining how to check blood pressure - talking about weight - talking about bowel movements - describing where pain is - describing what kind of pain one has
04	Giving Directions in and out of Buildings	1. Giving Patients Directions to Departments 2. Giving Visitors Directions to Patients' Rooms	- stating locations of places - giving directions - assisting visitors - asking for spellings of names - explaining how to ask for help
05	Examinations I	1. Taking Blood 2. Getting Urine and Stool Samples	- taking blood - providing comfort to patients - discussing conducting tests - describing how to provide urine and stool samples - explaining where to leave objects
06	Examinations II	1. MRI Scans 2. Ultrasound Scans	- conducting MRI scans - asking about personal possessions - giving instructions - conducting ultrasound scans - explaining the uses of things
07	Giving Orientation about Hospitalization	1. Describing Patients' Rooms 2. Answering Patients' Questions about Hospital Life	- describing the contents of rooms - explaining how to ask for help - talking about meals - talking about visiting hours - requesting changes in diets

08	Taking Care of Patients	1. Changing Patients' Dressings 2. Telling Patients to Change Positions	- asking how patients feel - changing dressings - describing wounds - instructing patients to change positions - explaining about bedsores
09	Discussing Medication	1. Explaining the Possible Side Effects of Medication 2. Answering Patients' Questions about Medication	- giving medication - describing side effects - explaining the purposes of medicines - answering questions about medication - explaining future actions with "let me"
10	Reassuring Patients and Guardians	1. Reassuring Patients Waking Up from Surgery 2. Reassuring Patients' Guardians	- greeting patients after waking up from surgery - asking how patients feel - describing the effects of anesthesia - speaking with guardians about patients' operations - providing reassurance to guardians
11	Discharging Patients	1. Informing Patients of Dos and Don'ts 2. Helping Patients Pay Their Bills	- discharging patients - giving medication to patients - reminding patients of what to do and what not to do - charging patients for their visits - discussing insurance
12	Handling Calls from Discharged Patients	1. Calls from Patients Who Need Something 2. Calls from Patients Who Are Complaining about Their Symptoms	- handling telephone calls describing problems - getting more information from patients - instructing patients to return to the hospital - asking patients about their symptoms - telling patients they will be called back soon

※ NCS(국가직무능력표준) 능력단위와의 연계성

분류	능력단위 및 분류번호	능력단위 요소	연계 Unit
직업기초능력 〉 의사소통능력	기초 외국어 능력 (A-2-마.)	외국어 듣기 일상생활의 회화 활용	UNIT 01-12
06. 보건·의료 〉 01. 보건 〉 02. 보건지원 〉 02. 병원안내	01. 환자응대관리 (0601020201_13v1)	진료 접수하기	UNIT 02
		환자진료정보 파악하기	UNIT 02 UNIT 03
		환자 배웅하기	UNIT 11
		환자 사후관리	UNIT 12
	03. 예약관리 (0601020203_13v1)	오프라인 예약 관리하기	UNIT 01
	04. 진료서비스지원관리 (0601020204_13v1)	진료 전 설명하기	UNIT 05 UNIT 06
	05. 환자상담관리 (0601020205_13v1)	전화 상담하기	UNIT 12
	06. 수납관리 (0601020206_13v1)	청구 수납하기 영수증 발행하기	UNIT 11

UNIT 01 Taking Reservations on the Phone

Warmup

다음은 병원 종사자들입니다. 각 병원 종사자의 업무를 아래에서 고르세요.

1. _____   2. _____   3. _____   4. _____

receptionist   surgeon   radiologist   nurse

- a. specializes in using X-rays, MRIs, and ultrasound
- b. does operations on patients
- c. helps patients make appointments with doctors
- d. helps people prevent diseases and improve their health

Vocabulary

주어진 의미에 어울리는 단어를 고르세요.

1. annual · · a. to make sure about something
2. confirm · · b. to wait
3. reschedule · · c. happening once a year
4. checkup · · d. to set for another time
5. hold on · · e. a physical examination

Warmup Listening

문장을 듣고 그에 맞는 대답을 고르세요.

1. _____
   a. I don't feel well.   b. Yes, I already saw him.
2. _____
   a. Today is Thursday.   b. That would be great.
3. _____
   a. No, it's not rescheduled.   b. No, I need to cancel it.

Conversation I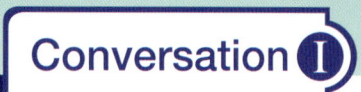

다음 대화를 듣고, 파트너와 함께 대화를 연습해 보세요.

Taking Reservations

Track 02

Receptionist	Good morning. Central Hospital. ¹How may I help you?
Patient	Hello. I'd like to make an appointment to see Dr. Min.
Receptionist	²What would you like to see him for?
Patient	I need to have my annual checkup soon. Are there any available times this week?
Receptionist	Yes, there are. ³What about this Friday at one in the afternoon? Dr. Min can see you then.
Patient	I'm afraid that's not a good time for me. Do you have anything open on Wednesday morning or Thursday afternoon?
Receptionist	Hold on a minute while I look . . . Ah, yes. How does Thursday at two thirty sound?
Patient	Perfect. I'd like to reserve that time, please. My name is David Murphy. I'm a patient of Dr. Min's.
Receptionist	Thank you very much, Mr. Murphy. See you on Thursday.

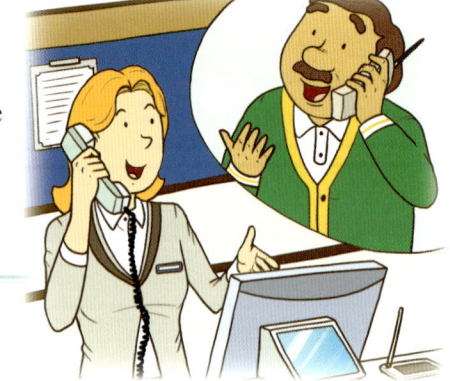

» Key Expressions

❶ How may I help you?   무엇을 도와 드릴까요?

환자에게 무엇을 도와 드리기를 원하는지 묻는 표현으로, 전화 응대 시 인사말로 자주 사용된다.

How may I be of service?   무엇을 도와 드릴까요?
How can I help you today?   오늘은 무엇을 도와 드릴까요?

❷ What would you like to see him for?   무슨 일로 의사 선생님을 뵈려고 하시지요?

환자에게 병원을 방문하려는 목적을 묻는 표현이다.

Why do you need to see the doctor today?   오늘 왜 의사 선생님을 뵈어야 하시지요?

❸ What about this Friday at one in the afternoon?   이번 주 금요일 오후 1시는 어떠세요?

What [How] about ~?을 사용하여, '~은 어떠세요?'라고 제안할 수 있다. 시각을 나타낼 때는 전치사 at을 사용한다.

How about any time after 3 PM on next Tuesday or Thursday?   다음 주 화요일이나 목요일 오후 3시 후에는 어떠세요?
How does next Monday, March 26, sound?   다음 주 월요일 3월 26일은 어떠세요?
Would this Thursday at 11 AM work for you?   이번 주 목요일 오전 11시 괜찮으세요?

Useful Phrases

전화 통화 중 상대방에게 잠시 기다려 달라고 요청하는 표현

Hold on a minute. 잠시만 기다려 주세요.

Please hold (the line). 끊지 말고 기다려 주세요.

One moment, please. 잠시만요.

12 | Taking Reservations on the Phone

Basic Drills

A 주어진 문장에 어울리는 대답을 고르세요.

1. How may I help you?
2. What about this Friday at one in the afternoon?
3. What would you like to see him for?

a. I need to have my annual checkup soon.
b. I'm afraid that's not a good time for me.
c. I'd like to make an appointment to see Dr. Min.

B 괄호 안의 말을 순서대로 배열하여, 주어진 의미를 영어로 표현하세요.

1. 무엇을 도와 드릴까요? (may / I / help / how / you)

_____

2. 무슨 일로 의사 선생님을 뵈려고 하시지요? (see him / would you / for / what / like to)

_____

3. 이번 주 금요일 오후 1시는 어떠세요? (this Friday / at one / about / what / in the afternoon)

_____

Buildup Activities

대화를 듣고 빈칸을 채운 후, 주어진 질문에 답하세요.

Receptionist	Good morning. Central Hospital. How may I be of (a)_____?
Patient	Hello. I want to make (b)_____ to see Dr. Hamilton.
Receptionist	Why do you need to see her?
Patient	I don't (c)_____ these days. Are there any available times today?
Receptionist	Yes, there are. What about today at (d)_____ in the morning? Dr. Hamilton has time then.
Patient	I'm sorry, but that's a bad time for me. Do you have anything available sometime in (e)_____?
Receptionist	Just a minute while I check . . . Ah, yes. How about this afternoon at (f)_____?
Patient	That would be great. I'll go there at that time. My name is Roger Martin. I'm one of Dr. Hamilton's patients.
Receptionist	Okay, Mr. Martin. See you later today.

1. Why does the caller want to see the doctor?
   a. He feels bad.　　　　　b. He broke his arm.　　　　　c. He need some medicine.

2. What time will the patient see the doctor?
   a. at eleven AM　　　　　b. at two thirty PM　　　　　c. at four fifteen PM

Conversation II

다음 대화를 듣고, 파트너와 함께 대화를 연습해 보세요.

Changing Reservations

Receptionist	Dr. Kim's office. How may I assist you?
Patient	Hi. My name is Karen Anderson. I have an appointment with Dr. Kim at eleven forty-five this morning.
Receptionist	That's correct, Ms. Anderson. ¹Are you calling to confirm your appointment?
Patient	Actually, I have to change it. I can't see the doctor because I have to visit a client.
Receptionist	I understand. ²Would you like to reschedule your appointment?
Patient	Yes, please. How about tomorrow morning at ten?
Receptionist	³He has an appointment then, but he doesn't have anything scheduled for eight thirty.
Patient	That's a bit early, but I think I can make it then. Thanks for your assistance.
Receptionist	You're welcome. Goodbye.

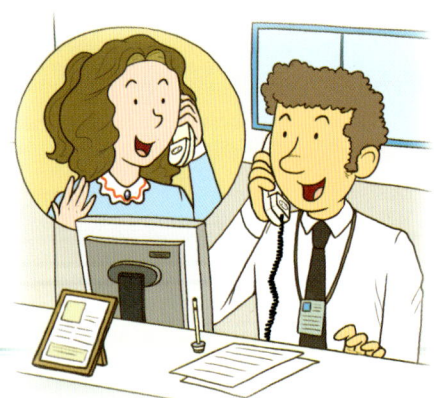

Key Expressions

❶ Are you calling to confirm your appointment?   예약을 확인하려고 전화하셨나요?

병원에 전화한 환자에게 예약 확인을 위해 전화했는지 묻는 표현이다.

Did you call to confirm your appointment?   예약을 확인하려고 전화하셨나요?

❷ Would you like to reschedule your appointment?   예약 일정을 변경해 드릴까요?

예약했던 시각에 내원할 수 없다는 환자에게 예약 일정을 변경하고 싶은지 물을 때 사용할 수 있다.

How would you like to reschedule your appointment?   예약 일정을 어떻게 변경해 드릴까요?

❸ He has an appointment then, but he doesn't have anything scheduled for eight thirty.

의사 선생님께서 그때는 예약이 있습니다만, 8시 30분에는 아무런 예약도 없습니다.

환자가 원하는 시각에 예약이 불가능한 경우, 진료가 가능한 시각을 안내할 때 사용할 수 있는 표현이다.

The doctor is not available this week, but she can see you anytime next Tuesday.
이번 주에는 의사 선생님께서 시간이 없으시지만, 다음 주 화요일에는 언제든 의사 선생님을 만나실 수 있습니다.

Useful Phrases

상대방의 감사 인사에 응답하는 표현

You're welcome. 천만에요.

It's my pleasure. 제 기쁨이지요.

Don't mention it. 별 말씀을요.

No problem. 괜찮습니다.

Basic Drills

A 주어진 문장에 어울리는 대답을 고르세요.

1. Would you like to reschedule your appointment? •   • a. That's a bit early, but I think I can make it then.
2. He doesn't have anything scheduled for eight thirty. •   • b. Actually, I have to change it.
3. Are you calling to confirm your appointment? •   • c. Yes, please.

B 괄호 안의 말을 순서대로 배열하여, 주어진 의미를 영어로 표현하세요.

1. 예약을 확인하려고 전화하셨나요? (you / calling / to confirm / are / your appointment)

   _____

2. 예약 일정을 변경해 드릴까요? (you / your appointment / like to / reschedule / would)

   _____

3. 의사 선생님께서 그때는 예약이 있습니다만, 8시 30분에는 아무런 예약도 없습니다.
   (but he doesn't have / anything scheduled / he has / then / for eight thirty / an appointment)

   _____

Buildup Activities

대화를 듣고 빈칸을 채운 후, 주어진 질문에 답하세요.

Track 05

Receptionist	Dr. Lee's office. Is there something I can help you with?
Patient	Hello. My name is Amy Butler. I am (a)_____ to see Dr. Lee at three o'clock this afternoon.
Receptionist	That's right, Ms. Butler. Do you need to see Dr. Lee before then?
Patient	No, I don't. In fact, I can't meet her today. I have to go (b)_____ right now.
Receptionist	I see. When is a (c)_____ for you to see the doctor?
Patient	How about tomorrow morning (d)_____?
Receptionist	Dr. Lee won't be here in the morning, but she will be here in the evening. (e)_____ five forty-five?
Patient	That's kind of (f)_____, but I have time then. Thanks for your help.
Receptionist	It's my pleasure. Have a nice day.

1. Why can't the caller see the doctor today?
   a. She has a meeting at work.
   b. She has to leave town.
   c. She has to take care of her son.

2. When will the caller see the doctor?
   a. this afternoon   b. tomorrow morning   c. tomorrow evening

Job Simulation I

A 〈보기〉에서 적절한 말을 찾아, 각 그림의 상황에 맞는 대화를 완성하세요.

> 보기
> I'd like to schedule an appointment with Dr. Min.
> How does this Thursday at two thirty sound to you?
> Why do you need to see the doctor?

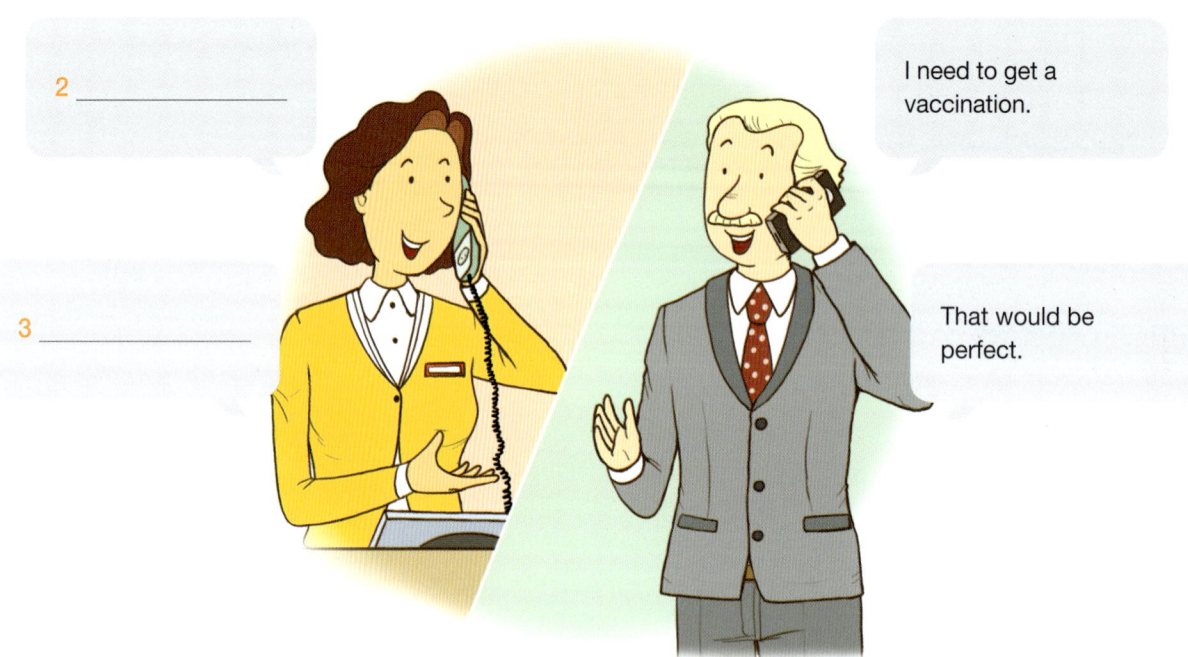

What can I help you with?

1. _____

2. _____

I need to get a vaccination.

3. _____

That would be perfect.

B 주어진 세 가지 상황을 이용하여, 파트너와 함께 각 상황에 맞는 대화를 연습해 보세요.

Situation	(a)	(b)	(c)
1	How may I help you	get my leg X-rayed	Tuesday morning at ten
2	How may I be of service	have a cast removed	tomorrow afternoon at three
3	How can I help you	see the doctor about my cough	this Thursday before noon

Receptionist   Good morning. Central Hospital. (a)_____?
Patient   Hello. I'd like to make an appointment to see Dr. Min.
Receptionist   What would you like to see him for?
Patient   I need to (b)_____. Are there any available times this week?
Receptionist   Yes, there are. What about (c)_____?

16 | Taking Reservations on the Phone

Job Simulation II

A 〈보기〉에서 적절한 말을 찾아, 각 그림의 상황에 맞는 대화를 완성하세요.

> 보기
> He's occupied then, but he's got an open slot at two fifteen.
> Did you call to confirm your appointment?
> Do you want to reschedule your appointment for another day?

1 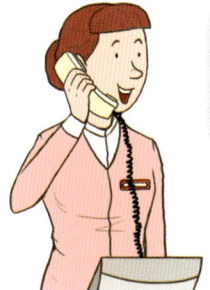 _____

Actually, I can't make it to my appointment today.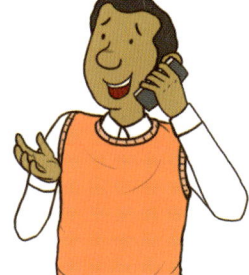

2 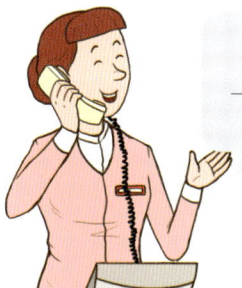 _____

Yes, I want to do that right now.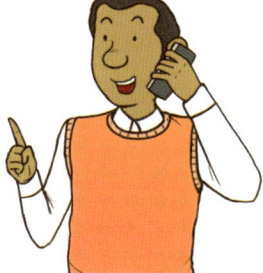

3 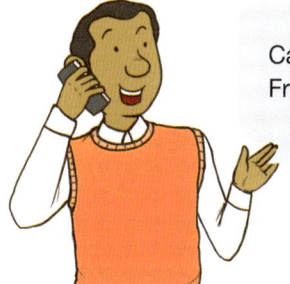 Can I see the doctor on Friday at one thirty?

_____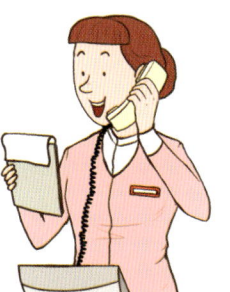

B 주어진 세 가지 상황을 이용하여, 파트너와 함께 각 상황에 맞는 대화를 연습해 보세요.

Situation	(a)	(b)
1	have to go to the airport	see the doctor at another time
2	need to see my dentist at that time	reschedule for later in the week
3	have a job interview	set up an appointment on another day

Receptionist Are you calling to confirm your appointment?

Patient Actually, I have to change it. I can't see the doctor because I (a)_____.

Receptionist I understand. Would you like to (b)_____?

Patient Yes, please.

Reading & Listening

다음 지문을 읽고, 음성을 들어 보세요.

The Origin of Nurses

Track 06

Doctors [1]have helped sick and injured patients for thousands of years. They have also had assistants. Those were the first nurses. However, those nurses had very little formal training. Most of them belonged to religious institutions and were monks or nuns. Modern nursing did not begin until the nineteenth century. During that time, war began to change. Because of modern weapons, large numbers of soldiers were wounded. These men often had no one to help them get better. Women such as Florence Nightingale and Clara Barton started taking care of those injured soldiers. They were the first modern nurses. As medical knowledge improved, nurses learned as well. They became able to take care of their patients better than ever. That allowed them to nurse their patients back to good health. In fact, that is why they are called nurses: because they nurse, or take care of, their patients and [2]help them get better.

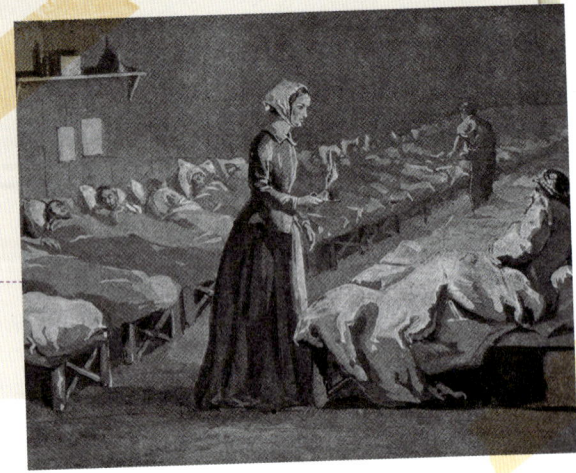

Words & Phrases

formal proper; official   **institution** an organization   **nun** a female monk
wounded injured; hurt   **improve** to get better

Basic Grammar

1 현재완료 have + p.p.

과거의 일이 현재에도 계속되고 있음을 나타낼 때, 또는 과거의 일이 현재에도 영향을 미치고 있음을 나타낼 때 현재완료를 사용한다.

Many doctors have treated him for a few months.   많은 의사가 몇 달째 그를 치료하고 있다.
As a nurse, Jane has worked at Seattle Hospital for over 10 years.   간호사로서, Jane은 Seattle 병원에서 10년 넘게 근무하고 있다.

2 help + 목적어 + (to) V   목적어가 ~하는 것을 돕다

help를 이용하여 '목적어가 ~하는 것을 돕다'라는 의미를 나타낼 수 있다. 이러한 경우, 목적격 보어 자리에는 to부정사가 올 수도 있고 동사원형이 올 수도 있다.

Would you help me (to) find the pediatric ward?   제가 소아과 병동을 찾는 것을 도와 주시겠어요?
The nurse helped the patient (to) get better.   간호사는 환자가 낫도록 도와 주었다.

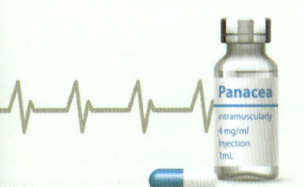

TIPS & TIPS

간호사라고 다 여자는 아니랍니다!

대다수의 간호사가 여자라는 사실 때문에, 사람들은 보통 간호사라고 하면 여자만 생각합니다. 하지만 남자 간호사도 있습니다. 과거에는 간호사가 모두 남자였던 적도 있었지요. 기원전 250년 인도에 처음 설립된 간호 학교에서는 여학생을 받지 않았습니다. 중세에도 남자 간호사가 많았습니다. 기사 역할과 간호사 역할을 동시에 하는 남자도 있었어요. 적과 싸우는 일도 하고 부상자를 치료하는 일도 했던 거지요. 1800년대에 들어서서야 지금처럼 여자 간호사가 많아졌답니다.

UNIT 02 Receiving Patients

Warmup
신체의 각 부위에 맞는 명칭을 오른쪽에서 찾아 써 보세요.

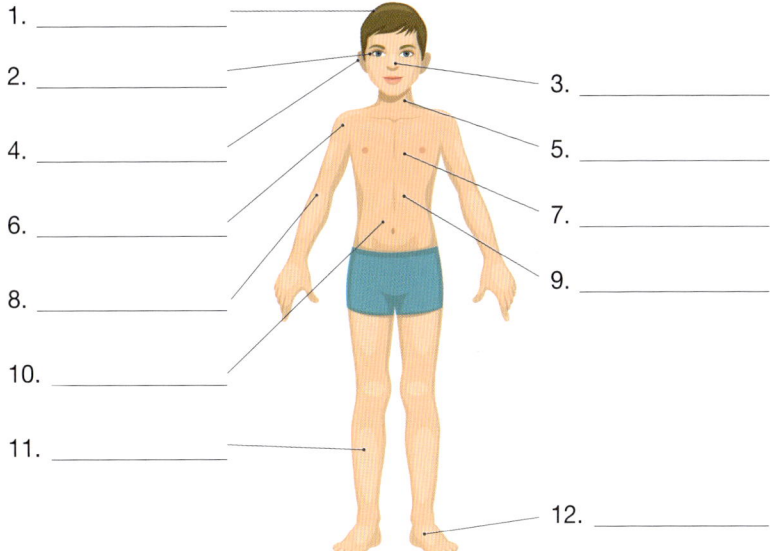

1. _____
2. _____
3. _____
4. _____
5. _____
6. _____
7. _____
8. _____
9. _____
10. _____
11. _____
12. _____

chest
neck
waist
eye
stomach
foot
ear
shoulder
head
nose
arm
leg

Vocabulary
주어진 의미에 어울리는 단어를 고르세요.

1. form • • a. an official paper; a sheet
2. sore • • b. a sign of a sickness
3. complete • • c. hurt; painful
4. symptom • • d. the regular beating of the heart
5. pulse • • e. to finish

Track 07

Warmup Listening
문장을 듣고 그에 맞는 대답을 고르세요.

1. _____
   a. Yes, I'm in the hospital.   b. No, I have been here before.
2. _____
   a. Sure. I can do that.   b. These are the forms.
3. _____
   a. For about two days.   b. Three days ago.

Conversation I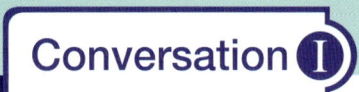

다음 대화를 듣고, 파트너와 함께 대화를 연습해 보세요.

Receiving Patients

Patient	Hello. My name is Tina Watson. I have an appointment with Dr. Kang at two o'clock.
Receptionist	Good afternoon, Ms. Watson. ¹Is this your first time to visit Dr. Kang?
Patient	Yes, it is. I've never been here before.
Receptionist	Okay. You need to fill out these forms, please. ²It should take about ten minutes.
Patient	No problem.
Receptionist	And I have to see your insurance card if you have one.
Patient	Here is my card.
Receptionist	Thank you. ³Why don't you complete the forms and bring them back when you're finished?
Patient	All right. I'll be back soon.

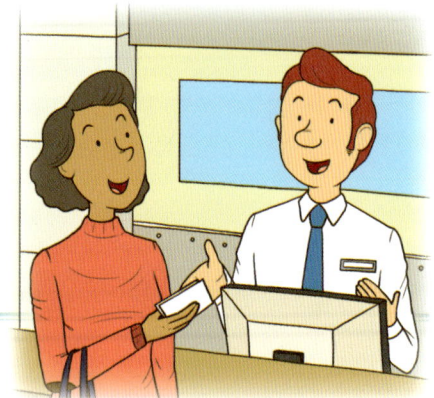

» Key Expressions

❶ Is this your first time to visit Dr. Kang?   강 선생님을 방문하시는 것은 이번이 처음이세요?

환자에게 초진인지 묻는 표현이다.

Is it your first time here?   이곳(이 병원)은 처음이세요?
Have you been here before?   전에 이곳(이 병원)에 오신 적 있으세요?

❷ It should take about ten minutes.   10분 정도 걸릴 겁니다.

'시간이 걸리다'라는 의미의 take를 사용하여, 시간이 얼마나 걸리는지 표현할 수 있다. 여기에서 should는 예상·추측을 나타내어 '~일 것이다'라는 뜻으로 쓰였다.

You should be done in about 5 minutes.   약 5분 후에 끝날 겁니다.
It usually takes fewer than 20 minutes.   보통 20분이 채 안 걸립니다.

❸ Why don't you complete the forms and bring them back when you're finished?

이 서식들을 작성하시고, 작성이 끝나시면 서식들을 다시 가져다 주시겠어요?

환자에게 서식 작성을 요청하는 표현으로, Why don't you ~?는 제안이나 권유를 할 때 사용하는 부드러운 표현이다. 서식이 하나인 경우에는 the form이라고 하면 된다.

Please bring back the forms once you are finished.   작성이 끝나시면 서식들을 다시 가져다 주세요.
Would you fill in [out] the forms first?   먼저 이 서식들을 작성해 주시겠어요?

Useful Phrases ➕

You need to V ~하셔야 합니다.

You need to fill out these forms. 이 서식들을 작성하셔야 합니다.
You need to show me your ID and insurance card. 저에게 신분증과 보험증을 보여 주셔야 합니다.
You need to make an appointment. 진료예약을 하셔야 합니다.
You need to talk to the doctor about that. 그것에 관해서는 의사 선생님과 이야기하셔야 합니다.
You need to wait another hour to see the doctor. 의사 선생님을 보시려면 한 시간 더 기다리셔야 합니다.

Basic Drills

A 주어진 문장에 어울리는 대답을 고르세요.

1. Is this your first time to visit Dr. Kang? •   • a. Yes, it is.
2. I have to see your insurance card if you have one. •   • b. All right. I'll be back soon.
3. Why don't you complete the forms and bring them back when you're finished? •   • c. Here is my card.

B 괄호 안의 말을 순서대로 배열하여, 주어진 의미를 영어로 표현하세요.

1. 강 선생님을 방문하시는 것은 이번이 처음이세요? (your first time / is / this / Dr. Kang / to visit)

   _____

2. 10분 정도 걸릴 겁니다. (about / should / it / take / ten minutes)

   _____

3. 이 서식들을 작성하시고, 작성이 끝나시면 서식들을 다시 가져다 주시겠어요?
   (and / bring them back / why don't you / complete the forms / when you're finished)

   _____

Buildup Activities

대화를 듣고 빈칸을 채운 후, 주어진 질문에 답하세요.

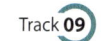

Patient	Hello. My name is Deanna Carpenter. I'm (a)_____ to see Dr. Simmons at ten thirty.
Receptionist	Good morning, Ms. Carpenter. Have you seen Dr. Simmons before?
Patient	No, I haven't. This is my (b)_____ to visit his office.
Receptionist	All right. Would you please (c)_____ these forms then? It will take around fifteen minutes.
Patient	Sure. I can do that.
Receptionist	And I need to see your (d)_____ card if you have it.
Patient	This is my (e)_____.
Receptionist	Thank you very much. How about (f)_____ all of the forms? Then, bring them back when you're done.
Patient	Okay. I'll be back in a bit.

1. How many times has the patient visited the office before?

   a. zero   b. one   c. two

2. What does the receptionist ask the patient to do?

   a. sign up for health insurance

   b. fill out some forms

   c. pay before seeing the doctor

Conversation II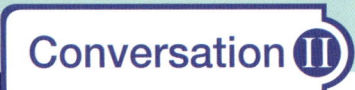

다음 대화를 듣고, 파트너와 함께 대화를 연습해 보세요.

Asking Patients about Their Conditions

Track 10

Nurse	Good morning, Mr. Morris. What's bothering you today?
Patient	I think I'm coming down with a cold. I feel terrible right now.
Nurse	I'm very sorry to hear that. What are your symptoms?
Patient	I've got a sore throat and a runny nose. My ears are plugged up. I think I have a temperature, too.
Nurse	Do you have any aches and pains? ¹Does your head hurt?
Patient	No, my head doesn't hurt, and neither does the rest of my body.
Nurse	Well, it doesn't sound bad then. ²How long have you had these symptoms?
Patient	I started to feel bad last night after I got home from work.
Nurse	Okay. ³Let me check your temperature and pulse. The doctor will be in to see you in just a few moments.

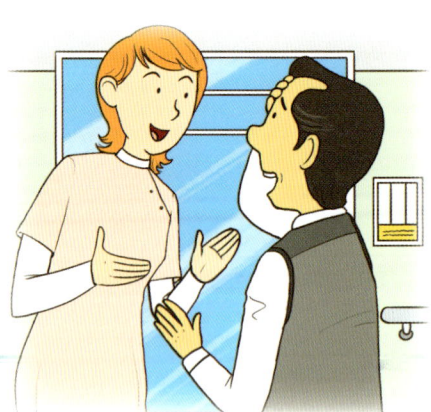

≫ Key Expressions

❶ **Does your head hurt?**   머리가 아프세요?

환자에게 두통이 있는지 묻는 표현이다. 다음 표현들도 환자에게 통증이나 불편감이 있는지 물을 때 사용할 수 있다.

Do you feel dizzy?   어지러우세요?
Do you have any rashes?   발진이 있나요?
Do you have any blood in your urine?   소변에 피가 비치나요?

❷ **How long have you had these symptoms?**   이 증상들을 겪은 지 얼마나 되셨나요?

환자가 겪고 있는 증상이 얼마나 되었는지 묻는 표현이다. had 대신 experienced를 쓸 수도 있다.

When did these symptoms start?   언제 이 증상들이 시작되었나요?

❸ **Let me check your temperature and pulse.**   체온과 맥박을 재 드리겠습니다.

환자에게 체온과 맥박을 재 주겠다고 말하는 표현이다.

I need to check your temperature and pulse.   체온과 맥박을 재야 합니다.

Useful Phrases

환자가 내원한 이유를 묻는 표현

What's bothering you today?   오늘은 어디가 아파서 오셨어요?
What brings [brought] you here?   이곳(병원)에는 어떤 일로 오셨어요?
What seems to be the problem?   어떤 문제가 있으세요?

Basic Drills

A 주어진 문장에 어울리는 대답을 고르세요.

1. What are your symptoms? •   • a. I think I'm coming down with a cold.
2. What's bothering you today? •   • b. I've got a sore throat and a runny nose.
3. How long have you had these symptoms? •   • c. I started to feel bad last night.

B 괄호 안의 말을 순서대로 배열하여, 주어진 의미를 영어로 표현하세요.

1. 머리가 아프세요? (head / does / your / hurt)
   _____

2. 이 증상들을 겪은 지 얼마나 되셨나요? (have you / how / long / these symptoms / had)
   _____

3. 체온과 맥박을 재 드리겠습니다. (me / temperature and pulse / check / your / let)
   _____

Buildup Activities

대화를 듣고 빈칸을 채운 후, 주어진 질문에 답하세요.   Track 11

Nurse	Hello, Mr. Thompson. What's the matter with you today?
Patient	I feel like I'm coming down with (a)_____. I feel awful right now.
Nurse	That's bad news. What (b)_____ do you have?
Patient	My (c)_____, and I've got a runny nose. My ears won't pop either. Lastly, I've got a slight fever.
Nurse	Do you have any aches and pains? Are you getting any (d)_____?
Patient	No, my head and the rest of my body are fine.
Nurse	Okay, that doesn't seem bad. When did these symptoms start?
Patient	I began feeling bad yesterday afternoon while I was (e)_____.
Nurse	All right. I need to check your (f)_____ and pulse . . . Dr. Kim will be here to see you in just a moment.

1. What is NOT wrong with the patient?
   a. He has a runny nose.
   b. His throat hurts.
   c. He has a headache.

2. When did the patient's symptoms start?
   a. this morning
   b. last night
   c. yesterday afternoon

Unit 02 | 23

Job Simulation I

A 〈보기〉에서 적절한 말을 찾아, 각 그림의 상황에 맞는 대화를 완성하세요.

> 보기
> May I see your insurance card?
> Yes, I am. I'm a new patient.
> All right. I'll be back in a few minutes.

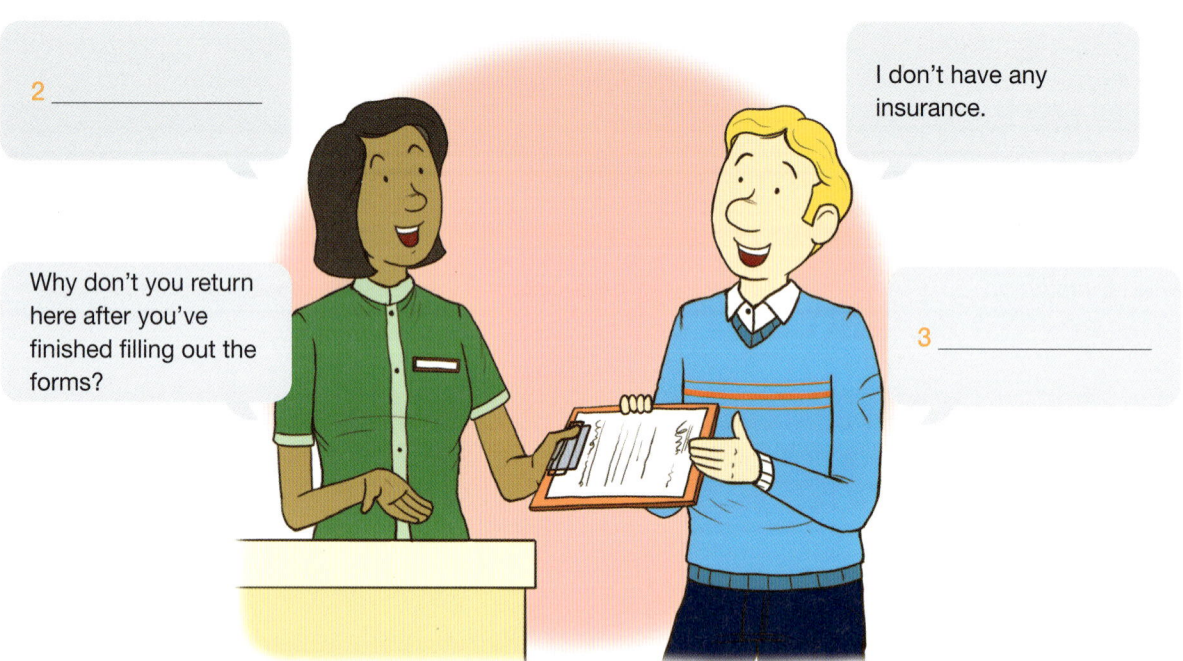

Are you visiting Dr. Lee for the first time?

1. _____

2. _____

I don't have any insurance.

Why don't you return here after you've finished filling out the forms?

3. _____

B 주어진 세 가지 상황을 이용하여, 파트너와 함께 각 상황에 맞는 대화를 연습해 보세요.

Situation	(a)	(b)
1	in this hospital	fill in these forms
2	to meet with Dr. Lee	complete these forms
3	to come to this office	fill out this form

Receptionist	Good afternoon, Ms. Watson. Is this your first time (a)_____?
Patient	Yes, it is. I've never been here before.
Receptionist	Okay. You need to (b)_____, please. It should take about ten minutes.
Patient	No problem.

Job Simulation II

A 〈보기〉에서 적절한 말을 찾아, 각 그림의 상황에 맞는 대화를 완성하세요.

> 보기
>
> For instance, do you have a headache?
> I have to check your temperature and pulse.
> I started to get sick this morning.

1

_____

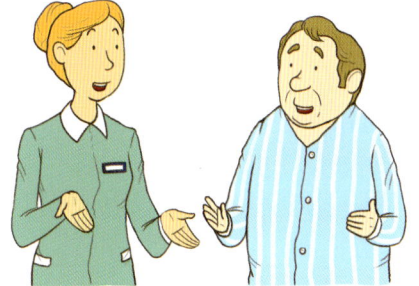

No, my head feels fine.

2

When did your symptoms begin?

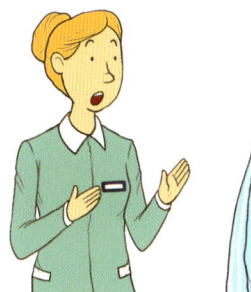 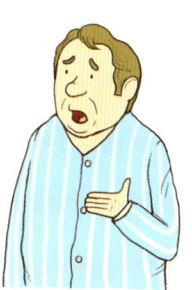

_____

3

What are you going to do next?

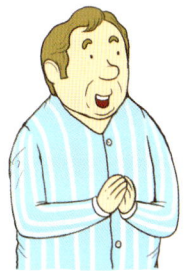 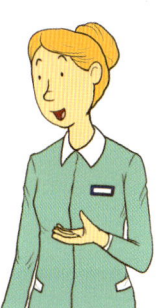

_____

B 주어진 세 가지 상황을 이용하여, 파트너와 함께 각 상황에 맞는 대화를 연습해 보세요.

Situation	(a)	(b)	(c)
1	I've got a temperature	Are you experiencing any pains	about three hours ago
2	I'm a bit feverish	Does any part of your body hurt	when I woke up this morning
3	I might have a fever	Is any part of your body hurting you	right before I went to bed last night

Patient   I've got a sore throat and a runny nose. My ears are plugged up. I think (a)_____, too.

Nurse   (b)_____? Does your head hurt?

Patient   No, my head doesn't hurt, and neither does the rest of my body.

Nurse   Well, it doesn't sound bad then. How long have you had these symptoms?

Patient   I started to feel bad (c)_____.

Reading & Listening

다음 지문을 읽고, 음성을 들어 보세요.

Various Types of Nurses

Track 12

Many people do not realize it, but there are several types of nurses. There are more registered nurses (RN) than any other kinds of nurses. RNs give medication, monitor patients' vital signs, and help treat patients. RNs work with doctors [1]when they examine and operate on patients, too. Licensed practical nurses collect samples from patients and monitor medical equipment. They also record information about patients and assist doctors and RNs when they conduct tests and do medical procedures. Nurse practitioners can diagnose illnesses and treat patients. They [2]may also write prescriptions for patients. Those are the three most common types of nurses. There are other nurses though. Nurse midwives are RNs who work with pregnant women. Certified registered nurse anesthetists specialize in anesthetics. They work closely with surgeons, dentists, and anesthesiologists. And home health nurses help take care of patients in their own homes.

Words & Phrases

monitor to watch carefully **vital signs** indicators of essential body functions such as temperature, pulse, and breathing **procedure** a method; an activity **prescription** written directions from a doctor regarding medicine a patient should take **anesthetics** a substance that causes part of the body to lose feeling

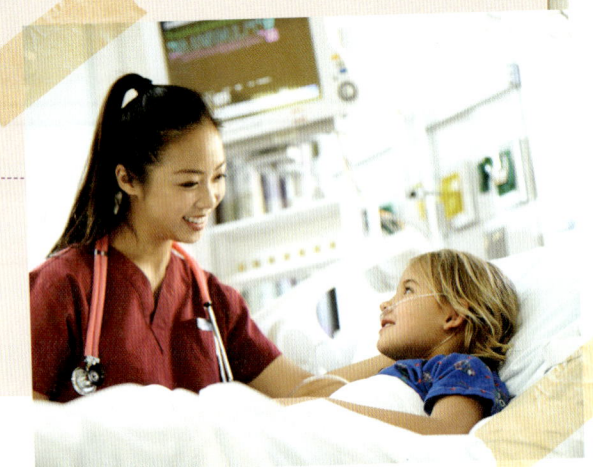

Basic Grammar

① 부사절을 이끄는 when

when은 의문사로서 '언제'라는 뜻을 나타낼 수도 있지만, 본문에서처럼 접속사로 사용되어 '~할 때'라는 시간의 의미를 나타내는 부사절을 이끌 수도 있다. while(~하는 동안)도 시간의 의미를 나타내는 부사절을 이끌 수 있다.

Please come to the counter when you are finished.   끝나시면 카운터로 오십시오.
You have to stay still while you are in the MRI machine.   MRI 기계 안에 계시는 동안에는 가만히 있으셔야 합니다.

② 가능성을 나타내는 may

조동사 may는 어떠한 행동이 일어날 수 있다는 가능성을 나타낸다. might와 could도 같은 의미로 사용될 수 있다.

The hospital might take walk-ins.   그 병원은 예약 없이 방문한 환자를 받을지도 모른다.
You could be discharged soon.   곧 퇴원하실 수도 있어요.

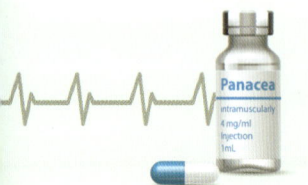

TIPS & TIPS

이거 사생활 침해 아니에요?

환자 입장에서는 가끔 간호사가 너무 사적인 질문을 한다고 느낄 수도 있습니다. 식습관부터 시작해서 담배는 피우는지, 술은 얼마나 마시는지 등 환자의 생활 습관에 대해 이것저것 물어 보니까요. 하지만 이런 질문을 하는 데는 그만한 이유가 있습니다. 현대인의 질병은 비만, 술, 흡연 같이 생활 습관과 관련된 경우가 왕왕 있기 때문인데요. 이러한 질문이 의료진으로서는 질병의 원인을 파악하는 데 도움이 되고 환자로서는 자신의 생활 습관에 대해 돌아 볼 기회가 되니, 마냥 불쾌해할 일만은 아니겠지요?

UNIT 03
Checking the Conditions of Patients

Warmup
다음 사진은 통증을 호소하는 환자들의 모습입니다. 각 환자가 느끼는 통증의 정도에 체크해 보세요.

My head hurts a little. But I think I can go to school today.

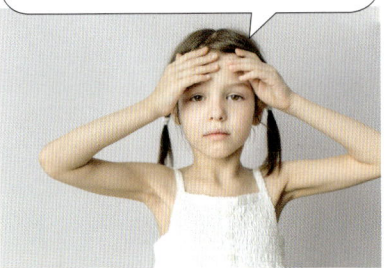

Ooh, my shoulder . . . I need to lie down and get some rest for a while.

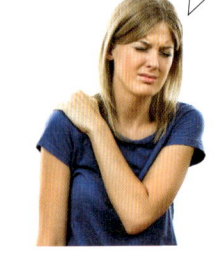

I can't stand this pain any longer! I'm going to call an ambulance right now!

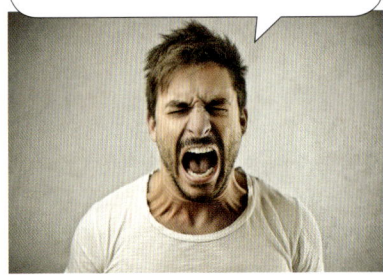

1. mild ☐
   moderate ☐
   severe ☐

2. mild ☐
   moderate ☐
   severe ☐

3. mild ☐
   moderate ☐
   severe ☐

Vocabulary
주어진 의미에 어울리는 단어를 고르세요.

1. put on weight •   • a. a part of the intestines
2. constant •   • b. a tool that measures weight
3. scale •   • c. severe; painful
4. bowel •   • d. continual; never ending
5. sharp •   • e. to become heavier

Track 13

Warmup Listening
문장을 듣고 그에 맞는 대답을 고르세요.

1. ▭
   a. Yes, I've lost 5 kilograms.   b. Yes, I've been eating a lot lately.
2. ▭
   a. No, it comes and goes.   b. Yes, it hurts.
3. ▭
   a. Right in my stomach.   b. A couple of hours ago.

Conversation I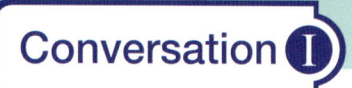

다음 대화를 듣고, 파트너와 함께 대화를 연습해 보세요.

Checking Patients' Conditions

Track 14

Nurse   I'm going to check your blood pressure. [1]Please roll up your sleeve and put your arm into the machine.
Patient   Should I press the button?
Nurse   Yes, please . . . Okay, your blood pressure is 110 over 80. That's normal. Now, [2]please step on the scale.
Patient   All right . . . I'm 72 kilograms.
Nurse   It looks like you've put on some weight recently. And [3]how many bowel movements do you have a day?
Patient   Usually 1 or 2 a day. But I've already been to the bathroom 4 times this morning.
Nurse   Are they loose?
Patient   No, they don't look bad.

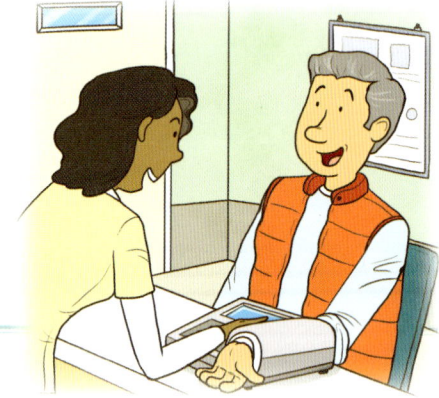

Key Expressions

❶ Please roll up your sleeve and put your arm into the machine.   소매를 걷고 팔을 기계 안에 넣어 주세요.

혈압을 재기 위해 환자에게 소매를 걷고 팔을 기계 안에 넣어 달라고 요청하는 표현이다.

Please put your arm into the machine and relax.   팔을 기계 안에 넣고 힘을 빼 주세요.

❷ Please step on the scale.   체중계에 올라서 주세요.

몸무게를 재기 위해 환자에게 체중계에 올라서 달라고 요청하는 표현이다.

Please take off your shoes and step on the scale.   신발을 벗고 체중계에 올라서 주세요.
What does the scale read?   체중계에 뭐라고 뜨나요?
How much do you weigh?   몸무게가 몇이세요?

❸ How many bowel movements do you have a day?   대변은 하루에 몇 번이나 보세요?

환자에게 하루에 몇 번 대변을 보는지 묻는 표현이다.

Have you had a bowel movement today?   오늘 대변 보셨어요?
Have you had any problems with your bowel movements?   배변 문제를 겪고 계시나요?
Do you have diarrhea or constipation?   설사나 변비가 있으세요?

Useful Phrases ➕

| It looks like ~   ~인 것 같네요. |

It looks like you've put on some weight recently. 요새 체중이 좀 느신 것 같네요.
It looks like you have lost some weight. 살이 좀 빠지신 것 같네요.
It looks like you haven't slept very well recently. 요새 잠을 잘 못 주무시는 것 같네요.
It looks like you need to see a specialist. 전문의에게 진료를 받으셔야 할 것 같네요.

Basic Drills

A 주어진 문장에 어울리는 대답을 고르세요.

1. I'm 72 kilograms. •   • a. Usually 1 or 2 a day.
2. Should I press the button? •   • b. It looks like you've put on some weight recently.
3. How many bowel movements do you have a day? •   • c. Yes, please.

B 괄호 안의 말을 순서대로 배열하여, 주어진 의미를 영어로 표현하세요.

1. 소매를 걷고 팔을 기계 안에 넣어 주세요. (your arm / into the machine / your sleeve / and / put / please roll up)

   _____

2. 체중계에 올라서 주세요. (scale / please / on / step / the)

   _____

3. 대변은 하루에 몇 번이나 보세요? (how many / have / a day / do you / bowel movements)

   _____

Buildup Activities

대화를 듣고 빈칸을 채운 후, 주어진 질문에 답하세요.

Nurse	I need to check your (a)_____. Would you please roll up your sleeve and put your arm into the machine?
Patient	All right. Do you want me to press the button?
Nurse	Yes, please . . . Okay, your blood pressure is 130 over 90. That's (b)_____. Next, how about stepping on the scale?
Patient	No problem . . . I'm (c)_____ kilograms.
Nurse	It looks like you've (d)_____ some weight recently. And how many (e)_____ do you have each day?
Patient	1 or 2. But I've already had to visit the bathroom (f)_____ this morning.
Nurse	Are they watery?
Patient	No, they look good.

1. What does the nurse say about the patient's blood pressure?

   a. It's low.

   b. It's normal.

   c. It's high.

2. How many times has the patient been to the bathroom this morning?

   a. 1 time

   b. 3 times

   c. 5 times

Conversation II

다음 대화를 듣고, 파트너와 함께 대화를 연습해 보세요.

Checking on Pain

Nurse: What brings you to the clinic today?
Patient: I have some awful pain in my belly.
Nurse: Can you tell me where it hurts?
Patient: Hmm . . . It's right here in the lower part of my stomach. It's mostly in the center, but sometimes the right side of my stomach hurts, too.
Nurse: I see. ¹Is the pain constant, or does it come and go?
Patient: It's a constant pain. ²It's very sharp, and it won't go away.
Nurse: When did the pain start?
Patient: About four hours ago. It wasn't too bad at first, but it is getting worse and worse. Do you think I've got appendicitis?
Nurse: It's too early to tell. ³The doctor will be here soon to examine you.

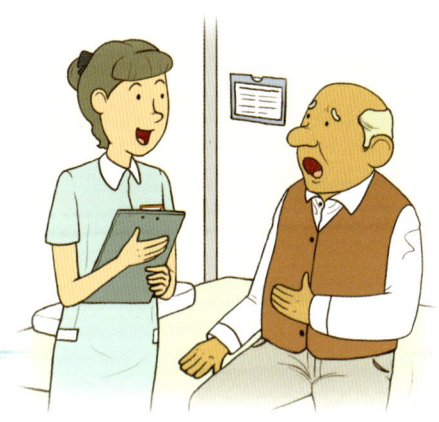

Key Expressions

❶ Is the pain constant, or does it come and go?   통증이 지속적인가요, 아니면 있었다 없었다 하나요?

환자가 겪는 통증의 빈도에 대해 물을 때 사용할 수 있는 표현이다.

How often do you feel the pain?   얼마나 자주 통증을 느끼세요?
Does the pain happen from time to time?   통증이 가끔 있으세요?

❷ It's very sharp, and it won't go away.   통증이 몹시 찌르는 듯 하고, 사라지지를 않아요.

통증의 종류 및 빈도를 묘사할 때 사용할 수 있는 표현이다.

I feel like I have pins and needles in my right arm.   오른팔에 저린 느낌이 있어요.
I feel the pain in my left knee all the time.   왼쪽 무릎에 통증이 계속 있어요.

❸ The doctor will be here soon to examine you.   의사 선생님께서 진찰하러 곧 이곳으로 오실 겁니다.

대기하고 있는 환자에게 의사가 곧 진찰하러 올 것이라고 할 때 사용할 수 있는 표현이다. soon 외에 in a moment 또는 shortly 등도 '곧'이라는 의미를 나타낼 수 있다.

The doctor will be with you in a moment.   의사 선생님께서 곧 오실 겁니다.
The doctor will be in to see you shortly.   의사 선생님께서 곧 오실 겁니다.

Useful Phrases

| 통증 부위를 설명하는 표현 |

It's right here in the lower part of my stomach.   바로 여기 아랫배예요.
The upper part of my right arm is sore.   오른쪽 팔뚝 윗부분이 아파요.
The pain under my shoulder blades is quite strong.   어깨뼈 아래 통증이 꽤 심해요.

Basic Drills

A 주어진 문장에 어울리는 대답을 고르세요.

1. Can you tell me where it hurts? • • a. It's right here in the lower part of my stomach.
2. When did the pain start? • • b. I have some awful pain in my belly.
3. What brings you to the clinic today? • • c. About four hours ago.

B 괄호 안의 말을 순서대로 배열하여, 주어진 의미를 영어로 표현하세요.

1. 통증이 지속적인가요, 아니면 있었다 없었다 하나요? (does it / constant / or / come and go / is the pain)
   _____

2. 통증이 몹시 찌르는 듯 하고, 사라지지 않아요. (it's / go away / and / it won't / very sharp)
   _____

3. 의사 선생님께서 진찰하러 곧 이곳으로 오실 겁니다. (you / here soon / the doctor / will be / to examine)
   _____

Buildup Activities

대화를 듣고 빈칸을 채운 후, 주어진 질문에 답하세요.

Track 17

Nurse	What brings you to the hospital today?
Patient	My (a)_____ really hurts.
Nurse	Can you tell me where it hurts?
Patient	Hmm . . . It mostly hurts in my (b)_____ stomach. It also hurts a bit on the left side of my upper stomach.
Nurse	I see. Does it feel (c)_____ all the time?
Patient	No, it's not constant. It's a (d)_____ pain, and it sometimes goes away.
Nurse	When did you feel the pain first?
Patient	Around noon. It wasn't that painful at first, but it has been (e)_____ since three o'clock. Do you think this is serious?
Nurse	I can't tell. The doctor will be here to (f)_____ you in a moment.

1. Where does the patient feel the most pain?
   a. in the lower stomach
   b. in the upper stomach
   c. in the bowels

2. What kind of pain is the patient experiencing?
   a. a continual pain
   b. a stabbing pain
   c. a mild pain

Job Simulation I

A 〈보기〉에서 적절한 말을 찾아, 각 그림의 상황에 맞는 대화를 완성하세요.

> 보기
> Around 1 or 2 normally.
> Your blood pressure is 140 over 90.
> Can you roll up your sleeve and put your arm into the machine, please?

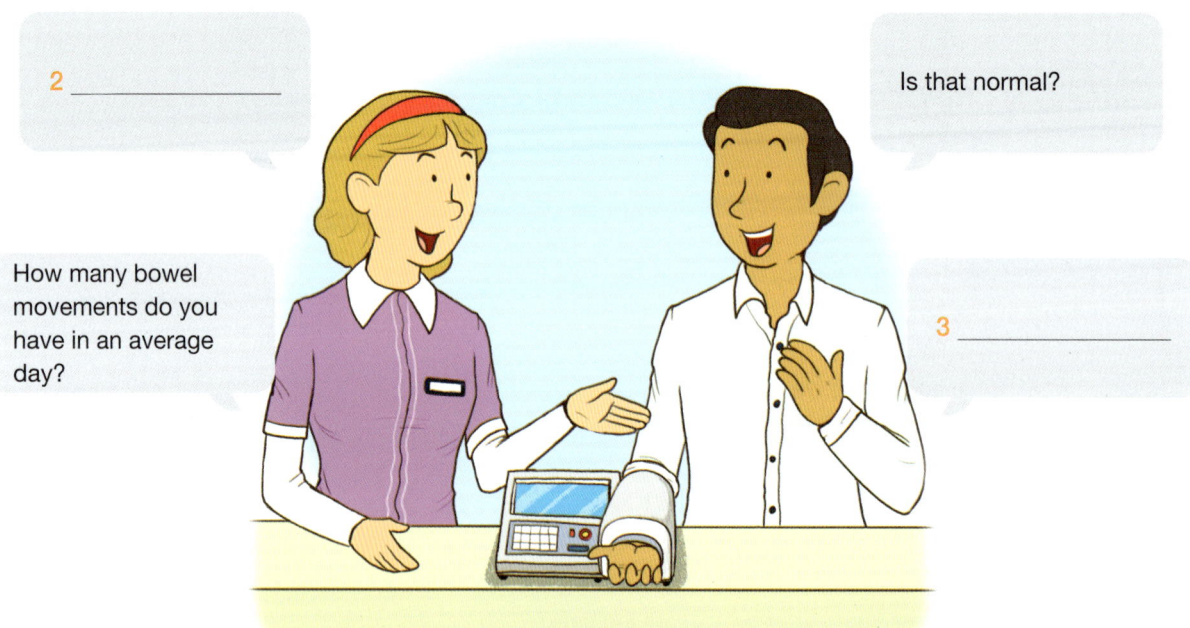

1. _____
   Okay. Do I need to press the button, too?

2. _____
   Is that normal?

How many bowel movements do you have in an average day?

3. _____

B 주어진 세 가지 상황을 이용하여, 파트너와 함께 각 상황에 맞는 대화를 연습해 보세요.

Situation	(a)	(b)
1	My weight is 64 kilograms	several times since last night
2	I weigh 58 kilograms	3 times in the past hour
3	My current weight is 83 kilograms	6 times today

Nurse   Now, please step on the scale.

Patient   All right . . . (a)_____.

Nurse   It looks like you've put on some weight recently. And how many bowel movements do you have a day?

Patient   Usually 1 or 2 a day. But I've already been to the bathroom (b)_____.

Checking the Conditions of Patients

Job Simulation II

A 〈보기〉에서 적절한 말을 찾아, 각 그림의 상황에 맞는 대화를 완성하세요.

> 보기
> It's a dull pain that won't go away.
> Yes, the pain is constant.
> I can't tell. Dr. Wilson will be with you in one moment.

1. Does it hurt all the time? 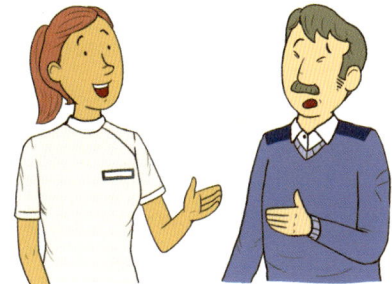 _____

2. Can you describe the pain for me? 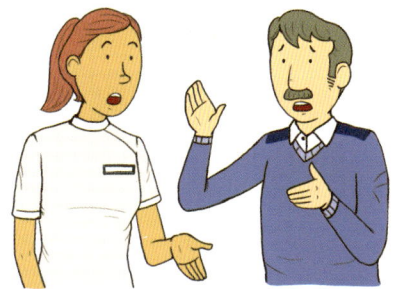 _____

3. Do you think I've got something serious? 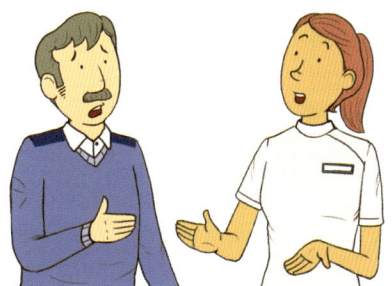 _____

B 주어진 세 가지 상황을 이용하여, 파트너와 함께 각 상황에 맞는 대화를 연습해 보세요.

Situation	(a)	(b)
1	Is the pain constant or intermittent?	a burning pain
2	Is the pain all the time, or does it come and go?	throbbing a lot
3	Is the pain steady or occasional	a shooting, aching pain

Patient I have some awful pain in my belly.

Nurse Can you tell me where it hurts?

Patient Hmm . . . It's right here in the lower part of my stomach.

Nurse I see. (a)_____?

Patient It's a constant pain. It's (b)_____, and it won't go away.

Reading & Listening

다음 지문을 읽고, 음성을 들어 보세요.

Pain Assessment Tools

Track 18

Patients often complain about pain. So nurses [1]must determine how badly they are hurting. One common pain assessment tool is the numeric scale for pain intensity. It runs from 0 to 10. Nurses ask patients to rate their pain on a scale from 0 to 10. 0 means that the patient is experiencing no pain. 10 means that the patient is experiencing the worst pain imaginable. The numbers 1-3 are for mild levels of pain, 4-6 are for moderate levels of pain, and 7-10 are for severe levels of pain. Another pain assessment tool is the Wong-Baker faces scale. Instead of numbers, it uses faces to assess pain. Nurses frequently use this with young children, but they can also use it with adults. There are 6 faces on the scale. A smiling face indicates no pain. [2]As the pain level increases, the face changes from a picture of someone frowning to a person crying in pain.

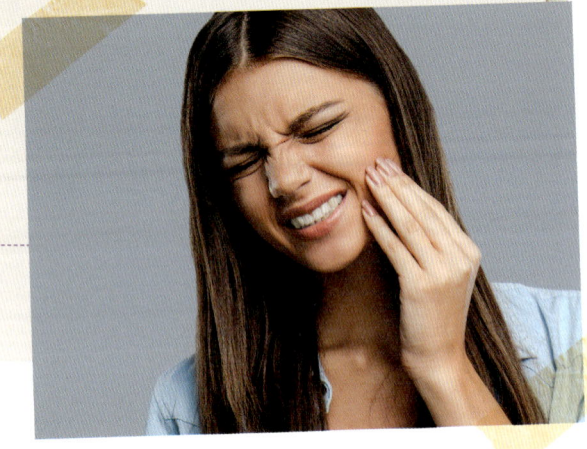

Words & Phrases

determine to learn; to find out **intensity** strength; power **imaginable** able to be thought **severe** serious **assess** to rate

» Basic Grammar

❶ '의무'를 나타내는 조동사 must

'(반드시) ~해야 한다'라는 뜻의 조동사 must는 어떤 행동에 대한 강한 의무를 나타낸다. have to도 의무의 의미를 나타낸다.

Nurses must keep their hands clean at work.   간호사는 일할 때 손을 청결히 유지해야 한다.
You have to follow the directions when you take medicine.   약을 복용하실 때는 지시사항에 따르셔야 합니다.

❷ 접속사 as

접속사 as는 여느 접속사와 마찬가지로 '주어 + 동사'를 이끌며, 본문에서는 '~하면서', '~할 때'의 의미로 쓰였다. 비슷한 의미의 접속사로는 while과 when이 있다.

As the pain medication started to work, the patient's condition got better and better.
진통제가 약효를 나타내기 시작하면서, 환자의 상태는 점점 더 나아졌다.

As the door opened, a nurse came in to the doctor's office.   문이 열리자, 간호사 한 명이 진료실로 들어왔다.

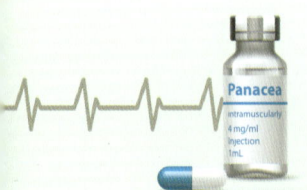

통증에도 종류가 있다고요?

간호사는 통증을 호소하는 환자를 상대해야 합니다. 하지만 모든 환자의 통증이 같은 것은 아닙니다. 통증은 급성통(acute pain), 만성통(chronic pain), 환상통(phantom pain) 그리고 방사통(radiating pain) 등으로 나눌 수 있지요. 급성통은 갑작스럽게 찾아와 시간이 지나면 사라지는 통증으로서, 부상을 입거나 수술을 받은 환자들이 흔히 겪는 통증입니다. 만성통은 6개월 넘게 지속하는 통증을 말합니다. 만성통을 겪는 환자는 계속되는 고통 탓에 우울하고 무력해지기 쉽습니다. 환상통은 절단 수술을 받은 환자가 겪기 쉬운 통증인데요. 신체의 어느 부위가 절단되어 실제로는 없어졌는데도, 환자는 그 부위에서 통증을 느낍니다. 방사통은 한 부분에서 다른 부분으로 전이되는 통증을 말합니다.

UNIT 04 Giving Directions in and out of Buildings

Warmup
다음은 치료나 검사가 필요한 환자들의 말입니다. 각 환자가 방문해야 할 진료과를 그림에서 고르세요.

1. "I had a car accident, and I need a CAT scan." _____
2. "I couldn't sleep last night because my skin itched." _____
3. "I have a kidney problem, so I need an operation." _____
4. "I can't breathe well. I think I have heart disease." _____

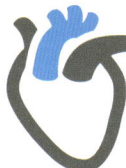 a Cardiology  b Radiology 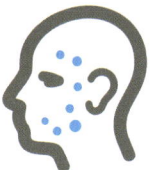 c Dermatology  d General Surgery

Vocabulary
주어진 의미에 어울리는 단어를 고르세요.

1. station • • a. a desk; a counter
2. spell • • b. directly; in a line
3. appointment • • c. to say the letters in a word correctly
4. lost • • d. a scheduled meeting
5. straight • • e. unable to find one's way

Warmup Listening
문장을 듣고 그에 맞는 대답을 고르세요.

Track 19

1. _____
   a. Yes, you're going to go there.   b. The Radiology Department is on the second floor.
2. _____
   a. M-A-R-K R-O-B-I-N-S-O-N.   b. It's Mark Robinson.
3. _____
   a. Go straight down the hall and then turn left.   b. It's five minutes away from here.

Conversation I

다음 대화를 듣고, 파트너와 함께 대화를 연습해 보세요.

Giving Patients Directions to Departments

Track 20

Patient: Pardon me, but could you give me some assistance, please?
Receptionist: I'll try. How may I help you, sir?
Patient: I'm looking for the Cardiology Department. I have an appointment with Dr. Lee, but I don't know where to go.
Receptionist: ¹The Cardiology Department is located on the fifth floor.
Patient: How can I get up there?
Receptionist: ²Do you see the elevators over there by the nurses' station?
Patient: Yes, I see them.
Receptionist: Take one of the elevators to the fifth floor. ³When you get off the elevator, turn left and walk straight down the hall. The Cardiology Department will be right in front of you.
Patient: Thank you so much for your assistance.

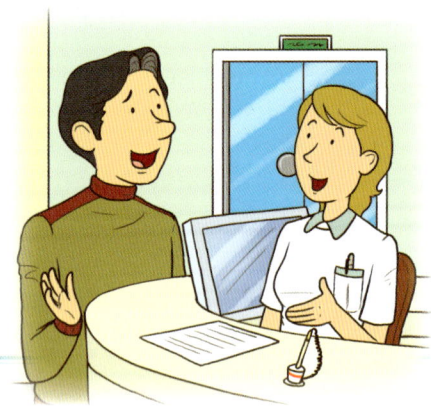

» Key Expressions

❶ The Cardiology Department is located on the fifth floor.   심장내과는 5층에 있습니다.

어떤 곳의 층수를 설명할 때는 be (located) on the ~ floor를 사용하여 '~ 층에 있다'라는 뜻을 나타낼 수 있다.

The cafeteria is on the third floor.   카페테리아는 3층에 있습니다.
We have a flower shop on the first basement floor.   지하 1층에 꽃집이 있습니다.

❷ Do you see the elevators over there by the nurses' station?   저쪽에 있는 간호사실 옆의 엘리베이터 보이세요?

길을 묻는 사람에게 길을 설명하는 과정에서 쓸 수 있는 표현이다. by는 '~ 옆에'라는 뜻으로 next to도 같은 의미로 사용할 수 있다.

Can you see the elevator next to the bathroom over there?   저쪽에 있는 화장실 옆의 엘리베이터 보이세요?

❸ When you get off the elevator, turn left and walk straight down the hall.
엘리베이터에서 내리시면, 좌회전하셔서 복도를 따라 직진하세요.

엘리베이터에서 내린 다음부터는 어떻게 가야 하는지 설명할 때 사용할 수 있는 표현이다.

After you get off the elevator, make a right turn. You will see room 405 on your right.
엘리베이터에서 내리신 다음, 우회전하세요. 오른쪽에 405호실이 보일 겁니다.

Useful Phrases ➕

무엇을 도와 드릴까요?

= How may [can] I help you?
= Do you need assistance?
= Can I help you with something?
= Is there something I can do for you?

Giving Directions in and out of Buildings

Basic Drills

A 주어진 문장에 어울리는 대답을 고르세요.

1. I'm looking for the Cardiology Department.
2. How can I get up there?
3. Could you give me some assistance, please?

a. How may I help you, sir?
b. Take one of the elevators to the fifth floor.
c. The Cardiology Department is located on the fifth floor.

B 괄호 안의 말을 순서대로 배열하여, 주어진 의미를 영어로 표현하세요.

1. 심장내과는 5층에 있습니다. (is / the Cardiology Department / the fifth floor / on / located)

2. 저쪽에 있는 간호사실 옆의 엘리베이터 보이세요? (the nurses' station / the elevators / over there / by / do you see)

3. 엘리베이터에서 내리시면, 좌회전하셔서 복도를 따라 직진하세요.
(down the hall / the elevator / and walk straight / when / you get off / turn left)

Buildup Activities

대화를 듣고 빈칸을 채운 후, 주어진 질문에 답하세요.

Track 21

Patient	Pardon me, but could you give me (a)_____, please?
Receptionist	I'll do my best. What do you need, ma'am?
Patient	I'm trying to find the maternity (b)_____. I am scheduled to meet Dr. Jeon in a few minutes, but I can't find my way there.
Receptionist	The maternity ward is on the (c)_____.
Patient	Can you tell me how I can get up there?
Receptionist	Sure. Do you see the (d)_____ over there by the ATM?
Patient	Yes, I see it.
Receptionist	Take it up to the third floor. Get off the escalator and (e)_____ to the end of the hall. The maternity ward will be (f)_____.
Patient	Thank you very much. You've been quite helpful.

1. What is the patient looking for?
   a. the Radiology Department
   b. the emergency room
   c. the maternity ward

2. How does the receptionist recommend going to the third floor?
   a. by walking up the stairs
   b. by taking the escalator
   c. by going up in the elevator

Conversation II

다음 대화를 듣고, 파트너와 함께 대화를 연습해 보세요.

Giving Visitors Directions to Patients' Rooms

Visitor	Hi there. My sister is a patient here, so I've come to visit her. Can you tell me where she is?
Receptionist	Of course. Can you give me her name, please?
Visitor	It's Karen Johnson.
Receptionist	¹How do you spell her last name?
Visitor	It's J-O-H-N-S-O-N.
Receptionist	Aha, I found her on the computer. ²Your sister is in room 322 in Building B. Right now, we're in Building A.
Visitor	Oh, I have to go to another building. How do I get there?
Receptionist	³Walk straight that way and go out the back door. Then, turn right. You'll see a tall blue building. That's Building B. Walk into it through the front door. You can take the elevator up to the third floor. If you get lost, ask a nurse there for help.
Visitor	I really appreciate it. Thanks a lot.

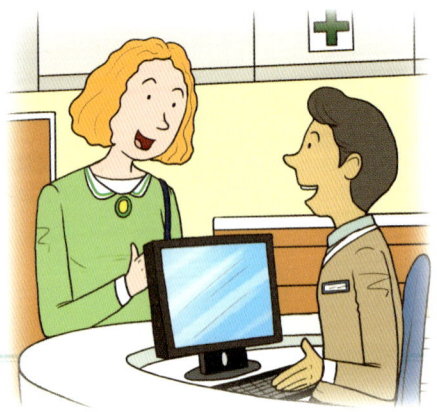

Key Expressions

❶ How do you spell her last name?   그분 성의 철자가 어떻게 되나요?
인적 사항을 정확하게 파악하기 위해 이름 등의 철자를 물어 볼 때 사용하는 표현이다
Could [Would] you spell that for me?   그것의 철자를 불러 주시겠어요?

❷ Your sister is in room 322 in Building B.   언니 되시는 분은 B동 건물의 322호실에 있습니다.
방문객에게 환자가 있는 병실을 알려 줄 때 사용할 수 있는 표현이다. 몇 호실인지는 room 뒤에 호수를 넣어 나타내며, 어떤 건물인지는 Building, Wing 등을 사용해 나타낼 수 있다.
Cardiology is in the West Wing.   심장내과는 서관에 있습니다.

❸ Walk straight that way and go out the back door.   저쪽으로 직진하셔서 후문으로 나가세요.
방문객이 가려는 병실이 다른 건물에 있는 경우 사용할 수 있는 표현이다.

Useful Phrases

> 그분(그 환자분)의 성함을 알려 주시겠어요?

= Can you give me her [his] name, please?
= May I have her [his] name, please?
= Could you tell me her [his] name?
= What's the name of the patient?

Basic Drills

A 주어진 문장에 어울리는 대답을 고르세요.

1. Can you give me her name, please? • • a. It's Karen Johnson.
2. How do you spell her last name? • • b. It's J-O-H-N-S-O-N.
3. How do I get there? • • c. Walk straight that way and go out the back door.

B 괄호 안의 말을 순서대로 배열하여, 주어진 의미를 영어로 표현하세요.

1. 그분 성의 철자가 어떻게 되나요? (spell / how / you / her last name / do)
   _____

2. 언니 되시는 분은 B동 건물의 322호실에 있습니다. (is / your sister / in Building B / room 322 / in)
   _____

3. 저쪽으로 직진하셔서 후문으로 나가세요. (go out / that way / and / the back door / walk straight)
   _____

Buildup Activities

대화를 듣고 빈칸을 채운 후, 주어진 질문에 답하세요.

Track 23

Visitor	Good evening. (a)_____ is hospitalized here, so I'm visiting her. Could you please tell me what room she is in?
Receptionist	I sure can. What's her (b)_____?
Visitor	It's Amelia Smith.
Receptionist	How do you (c)_____ her first name?
Visitor	It's A-M-E-L-I-A.
Receptionist	Aha, here she is. You can find her in room 503 in (d)_____. In case you don't know, we're in Building 1.
Visitor	Oh, she's in another building. Where is it?
Receptionist	Walk out the (e)_____ of this building. After that, take a left. You'll see a very tall white building. That's Building 3. Go right into it through the front door and take the elevator to the (f)_____. A nurse can help you if you can't find your way.
Visitor	Thanks for all your help. I appreciate it.

1. Who does the visitor want to see?
   a. his mother   b. his aunt   c. his sister

2. How should the visitor go out Building 1?
   a. through the front door
   b. through the back door
   c. through the side door

Job Simulation I

A 〈보기〉에서 적절한 말을 찾아, 각 그림의 상황에 맞는 대화를 완성하세요.

> 보기
> Can you see the elevators next to the nurses' station?
> I'm not sure where I should go.
> When you get off the elevator, turn right and walk about 30 meters.

1 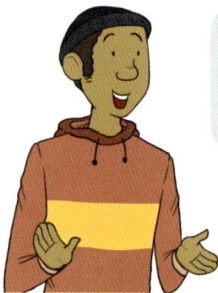 _____

The Radiology Department is on the second floor.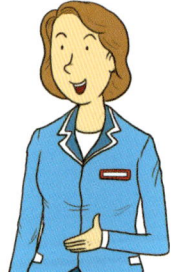

2 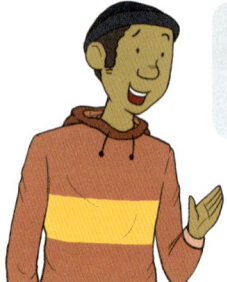 How can I get up to that floor?

_____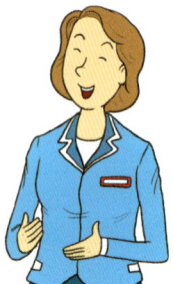

3 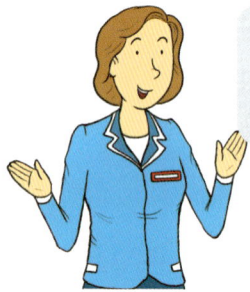 _____

Thank you very much for all your help.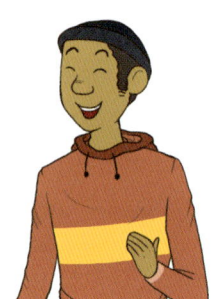

B 주어진 세 가지 상황을 이용하여, 파트너와 함께 각 상황에 맞는 대화를 연습해 보세요.

Situation	(a)	(b)	(c)
1	provide me with some assistance	there in 10 minutes	can be found on the second floor
2	help me out	with a doctor there	is on the third floor
3	lend me a hand	with Dr. Lee at 4:15	is on the tenth floor

Patient: Pardon me, but could you (a)_____, please?

Receptionist: I'll try. How may I help you, sir?

Patient: I'm looking for the Cardiology Department. I have an appointment (b)_____, but I don't know where to go.

Receptionist: The Cardiology Department (c)_____.

Job Simulation II

A 〈보기〉에서 적절한 말을 찾아, 각 그림의 상황에 맞는 대화를 완성하세요.

> 보기
> Walk that way and head out the back door.
> Your mother is hospitalized in room 912 in Building 5.
> Can you please tell me her name?

1. I'm here to visit my mother. 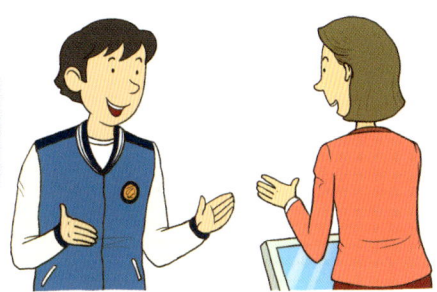 _____

2. _____ 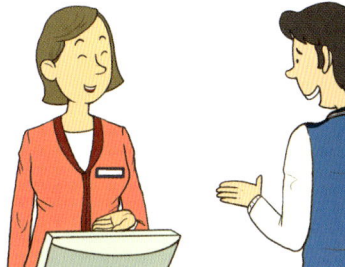 Oh, she's in a different building.

3. How can I get to that building? 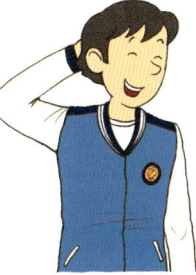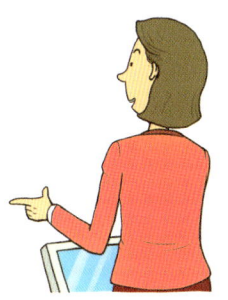 _____

B 주어진 세 가지 상황을 이용하여, 파트너와 함께 각 상황에 맞는 대화를 연습해 보세요.

Situation	(a)	(b)	(c)
1	on the third floor of Building B	Head in that direction	use the escalator to get to the third floor
2	staying in room 602 in Building B	Walk past the escalators	ride in the elevator to get to the sixth floor
3	in room 205 in Building B	Go that way	take the stairs to the second floor

Receptionist: Your sister is (a)_____. Right now, we're in Building A.

Visitor: Oh, I have to go to another building. How do I get there?

Receptionist: (b)_____ and go out the back door. Then, turn right. You'll see a tall blue building. That's Building B. You can (c)_____. If you get lost, ask a nurse there for help.

Reading & Listening

다음 지문을 읽고, 음성을 들어 보세요.

Various Departments in General Hospitals

Track 24

Most hospitals have the following areas: emergency rooms, operating rooms, intensive care unit (ICU), radiology, and maternity. Doctors examine patients in emergency rooms and conduct surgery in operating rooms. The ICU is for patients [1]with very serious conditions. Patients get X-rays in the Radiology Department, and the maternity ward is for pregnant women and mothers. General hospitals treat patients with all kinds of problems, so they have many other departments. Cardiology is for patients with heart problems. Geriatrics is for the elderly, and Dermatology is for skin care. Oncology is for patients with cancer, and Psychiatry is for people with mental issues. Ophthalmology is for eye problems, and Infectious Diseases is for dangerous viruses and illnesses. Some other common departments are Rheumatology, Urology, Hematology, and Neurology. The doctors and nurses in these departments work hard to give their patients the best care [2]possible.

Words & Phrases

pregnant woman a woman who is carrying a baby inside her body
treat to take care of a patient   **the elderly** old people   **mental** relating to the mind or brain   **issue** a problem

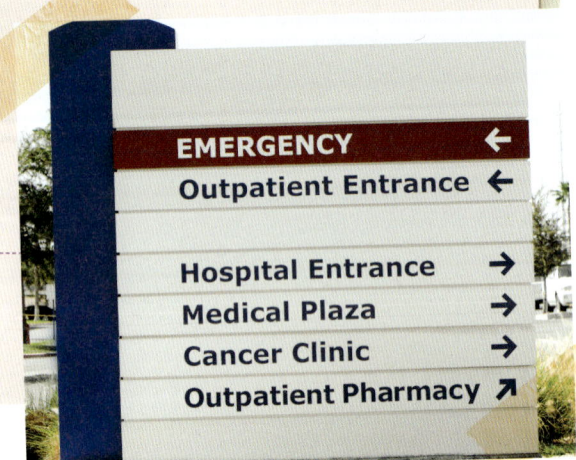

Basic Grammar

❶ '소유'를 나타내는 전치사 with

전치사 with에는 여러 가지 의미가 있으며, 본문에서는 '~이 있는', '~을 가지고 있는'이라는 '소유'의 의미로 쓰였다. 특히 병이 '있는', 즉 병에 걸린 상태를 나타내기 위해 with가 사용되었다.

People with cancer go to Oncology.   암에 걸린 사람들은 종양학과에 간다.
Young patients with serious illnesses stay in this ward.   중병에 걸린 어린 환자들은 이 병동에 머문다.

❷ -ible, -able로 끝나는 형용사

본문의 possible과 같이 -ible이나 -able로 끝나는 형용사는 명사를 뒤에서도 꾸며 줄 수 있다.

The hospital gave him the best treatment imaginable.   병원은 그에게 상상할 수 있는 최고의 치료를 제공했다.

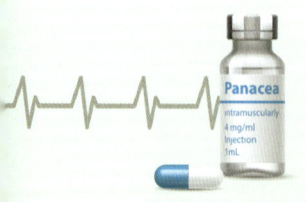

TIPS & TIPS

여기가 병원이야, 호텔이야?

과거에는 병원이라고 하면 진료실과 대기실 정도만 생각했지만, 요즘 종합병원은 그 이상을 보여 줍니다. 병원 의료진과 방문객을 위한 식당과 휴게실뿐만 아니라 커피숍, 은행과 서점도 흔히 찾아 볼 수 있습니다. 게다가 제과점, 꽃집, 편의점도 있지요. 병원에서 오랜 시간을 보내는 이들을 위해 병원에서 모든 것을 해결할 수 있도록 편의시설을 갖춘 것입니다. 그뿐인가요? 병원 안에서도 종교 활동을 할 수 있도록 원목실이나 법당 등이 마련된 병원도 있습니다. 심지어는 병원에서 문화생활도 누릴 수 있는데요. 외출이 어려운 입원 환자나 보호자를 위해 병원에서 음악회 등의 공연이나 미술 전시가 열리기도 합니다. 청진기를 목에 두른 의료진만 아니면 여기가 병원인지 호텔인지 헷갈릴 때도 있답니다!

UNIT 05 Examinations I

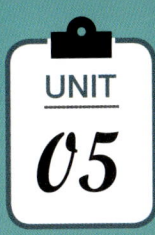

Warmup
다음은 검사 중에 간호사가 환자에게 요청할 수 있는 행동입니다. 각 사진에 해당하는 행동을 아래에서 찾아 써 보세요.

1. _____
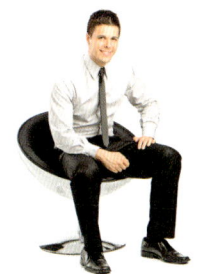

2. _____
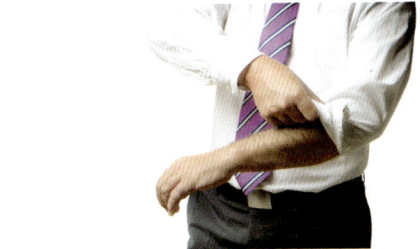

3. _____
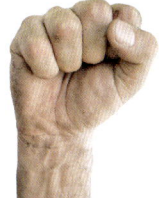

4. _____
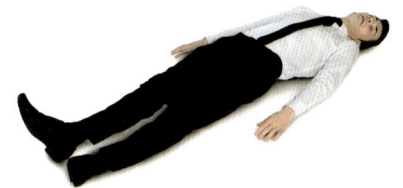

| roll up one's sleeve | take a seat | lie down | make a fist |

Vocabulary
주어진 의미에 어울리는 단어를 고르세요.

1. container   •   • a. solid waste from the body; feces
2. draw   •   • b. to take; to remove
3. urinate   •   • c. a cup; a bottle
4. fist   •   • d. to remove liquid waste from the body
5. stool   •   • e. a closed hand

Track 25

Warmup Listening
문장을 듣고 그에 맞는 대답을 고르세요.

1. _____
   a. That hurt a lot. b. Will this hurt?
2. _____
   a. This is a urine sample. b. You need to provide a urine sample.
3. _____
   a. Please get some urine in the container. b. Why don't you buy a smaller container?

Conversation I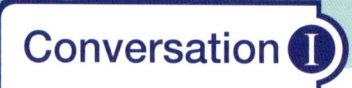

다음 대화를 듣고, 파트너와 함께 대화를 연습해 보세요.

Taking Blood

Track 26

Nurse	The doctor ordered me to run some blood tests today. ¹I'll draw some blood from you.
Patient	Is this going to hurt? I don't like having my blood taken.
Nurse	Don't worry about a thing. Now, please take a seat in this chair and roll up the sleeve on your left arm.
Patient	All right. What should I do next?
Nurse	²Please make a fist with your left hand and just relax. You may turn your head to the wall. Okay, ³you might feel a little sting . . . That's it. We're all done. You can open your hand now. Good . . . Let me put a bandage on your arm. How do you feel?
Patient	I don't feel well. I feel a bit dizzy.
Nurse	You should lie down for a moment. Here you go. You'll feel better soon.
Patient	Thanks.

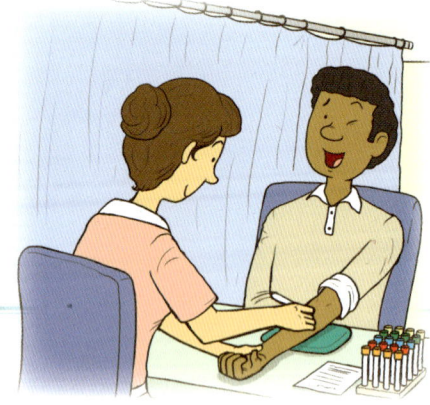

Key Expressions

① I'll draw some blood from you. 피를 좀 뽑겠습니다.

환자에게 혈액 검사를 위해 채혈을 하겠다고 안내하는 표현이다.

I need to take some blood from you. 피를 좀 뽑아야겠습니다.

② Please make a fist with your left hand and just relax. 왼손으로 주먹을 쥐시고 힘 빼세요.

이 표현은 채혈 시 환자에게 주먹을 쥐라고 할 때 사용할 수 있다.

Please hold out your right arm and make a fist. 오른팔을 내미시고 주먹을 쥐세요.

③ You might feel a little sting. 약간 따끔하실 수 있습니다.

환자가 마음의 준비를 할 수 있도록, 주삿바늘을 환자의 팔에 찔러 넣기 전에 쓸 수 있는 표현이다.

You will feel a little pinch. 조금 따끔하실 겁니다.

I'm going to inject this into your muscle, so you might feel some pain there.
근육에 이 주사를 놓을 거라서, 근육이 약간 뻐근하실 수 있습니다.

Useful Phrases

어떠세요? [괜찮으세요?]

= How do you feel?
= How are you feeling?
= Are you all right?
= Do you feel okay?

Basic Drills

A 주어진 문장에 어울리는 대답을 고르세요.

1. Is this going to hurt? • • a. Please make a fist with your left hand and just relax.
2. How do you feel? • • b. I feel a bit dizzy.
3. What should I do next? • • c. Don't worry about a thing.

B 괄호 안의 말을 순서대로 배열하여, 주어진 의미를 영어로 표현하세요.

1. 피를 좀 뽑겠습니다. (I'll / some blood / draw / from / you)

   _____

2. 왼손으로 주먹을 쥐시고 힘 빼세요. (with / and / please make a fist / just relax / your left hand)

   _____

3. 약간 따끔하실 수 있습니다. (a / little / might / you / feel / sting)

   _____

Buildup Activities

대화를 듣고 빈칸을 채운 후, 주어진 질문에 답하세요.   Track **27**

Nurse	The doctor asked me to run some (a)_____ on you today. So I have to take some blood.
Patient	Will this hurt? I don't like (b)_____ very much.
Nurse	You don't need to worry at all. Would you please sit down and (c)_____ your right arm?
Patient	No problem. What do you want me to do next?
Nurse	Make a fist with your right hand. Then, just sit back and relax. You can close your eyes if you want. You'll barely feel anything . . . All right. I'm all finished. I'll put this (d)_____ on your arm. Do you feel all right?
Patient	No, I don't. I feel a little (e)_____ now.
Nurse	You'd better (f)_____ for a minute. You can lie down here. You'll be as good as new in no time.
Patient	Thanks.

1. What does the patient dislike?

   a. needles   b. doctors   c. blood

2. What does the nurse tell the patient to do?

   a. go back to the waiting room

   b. lie down

   c. breathe deeply

Conversation II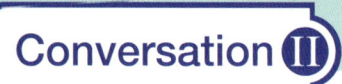

다음 대화를 듣고, 파트너와 함께 대화를 연습해 보세요.

Getting Urine and Stool Samples

Nurse: Dr. White isn't sure what's wrong with you. So we have to conduct some tests. ¹We need a urine sample and a stool sample.
Patient: I don't have to urinate right now.
Nurse: That's fine. Why don't you drink some water and wait a few minutes? . . . Okay, Mr. Taylor. Do you think you're ready?
Patient: I'll try now.
Nurse: ²Please get some urine in this container and stool in the other one. You may use the bathroom right here.
Patient: Should I bring these back to you?
Nurse: No. There's a cabinet in the bathroom. Please put them in there. ³Make sure the labels on the containers are facing outward.
Patient: Sure. I'll be back in a few minutes.

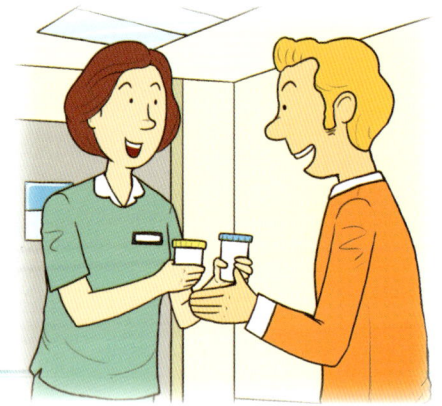

» Key Expressions

❶ **We need a urine sample and a stool sample.**   소변 샘플과 대변 샘플이 필요합니다.
이 표현은 대·소변 검사를 위해 환자에게 소변 및 대변 샘플이 필요하다고 말할 때 사용한다.
We need to collect urine and stool samples from you.   소변과 대변 샘플을 채취해야 합니다.

❷ **Please get some urine in this container and stool in the other one.**
이 통에는 소변을 담으시고 다른 통에는 대변을 담으세요.
환자에게 소변과 대변을 각각 어떤 통에 담아야 하는지 설명하는 표현이다.
Use this one for a urine sample and the other one for a stool sample.   이것은 소변 샘플에 다른 것은 대변 샘플에 사용하세요.

❸ **Make sure the labels on the containers are facing outward.**   반드시 통의 라벨이 바깥쪽을 향하도록 해 주세요.
Make [Be] sure ~는 '반드시 ~해라'라는 뜻으로, 환자에게 어떠한 지시나 당부를 할 때 사용할 수 있다.
Be sure to use the correct containers.   반드시 올바른 통을 사용해 주세요.
Make sure that you leave the cups in the cabinet.   반드시 컵을 캐비닛에 안에 두세요.

Useful Phrases

금방 올게요.

= I'll be back in a few minutes.
= I'll be back in a bit.
= I'll be right back.
= I'll come back in no time.

Basic Drills

A 주어진 문장에 어울리는 대답을 고르세요.

1. Should I bring these back to you?
2. We need a urine sample and a stool sample.
3. Make sure the labels on the containers are facing outward.

a. I don't have to urinate right now.
b. Sure. I'll be back in a few minutes.
c. No. There's a cabinet in the bathroom. Please put them in there.

B 괄호 안의 말을 순서대로 배열하여, 주어진 의미를 영어로 표현하세요.

1. 소변 샘플과 대변 샘플이 필요합니다. (a stool sample / we / a urine sample / and / need)

2. 이 통에는 소변을 담으시고 다른 통에는 대변을 담으세요.
   (in the other one / some urine / please get / and / stool / in this container)

3. 반드시 통의 라벨이 바깥쪽을 향하도록 해 주세요. (outward / the labels / on the containers / make sure / are facing)

Buildup Activities

대화를 듣고 빈칸을 채운 후, 주어진 질문에 답하세요.

Nurse: Dr. Yoon doesn't know what's wrong with you yet. So we have to run a few tests. We have to get a urine sample and a (a)_____ from you.

Patient: I just went to the bathroom ten minutes ago. I can't (b)_____ right now.

Nurse: That's fine. How about drinking (c)_____ and waiting a few minutes then? . . . Okay, Mr. Simpson, are you ready? Take these two containers to the bathroom. Please urinate in this one and defecate in the other one. The bathroom is down the hall on the left.

Patient: Do you want me to bring the (d)_____ back here?

Nurse: Please don't. There's a (e)_____ in the bathroom. You can put the containers in it. Just be sure the (f)_____ with your name on them are facing outward.

Patient: Okay. I'll be back here in a bit.

1. What did the man do ten minutes ago?
   a. He got a shot.
   b. He filled out some forms.
   c. He went to the bathroom.

2. What is on the label on each container?
   a. the patient's name
   b. the patient's ID number
   c. the patient's blood type

Job Simulation I

A 〈보기〉에서 적절한 말을 찾아, 각 그림의 상황에 맞는 대화를 완성하세요.

> 보기
> This might sting a bit.
> I need to get some blood from you.
> Could you please make a fist with your left hand and relax?

1
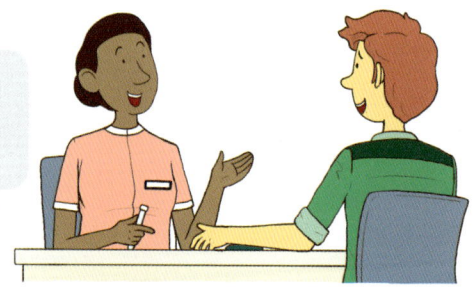
_____
Will this hurt a lot?

2
What would you like me to do?
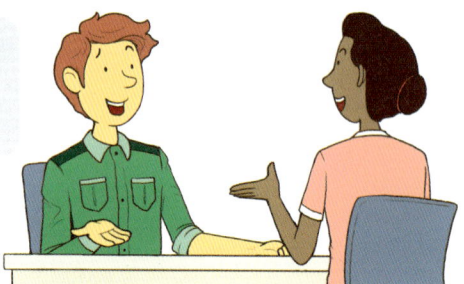
_____

3
_____
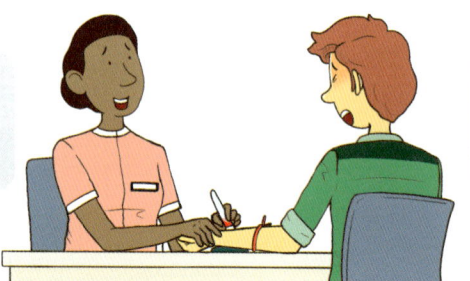
Ouch. I don't feel well.

B 주어진 세 가지 상황을 이용하여, 파트너와 함께 각 상황에 맞는 대화를 연습해 보세요.

Situation	(a)	(b)	(c)
1	you may feel something	I feel a bit dizzy	I think you should lie down
2	this might sting a bit	I feel a little lightheaded	You ought to lie back
3	this won't hurt a bit	My head is spinning	I want you to lie down

Nurse　Please make a fist with your left hand and just relax . . . Okay, (a)_____ . . . That's it. We're all done. Let me put a bandage on your arm. How do you feel?

Patient　I don't feel well. (b)_____.

Nurse　(c)_____ for a moment. You'll feel better soon.

Job Simulation II

A 〈보기〉에서 적절한 말을 찾아, 각 그림의 상황에 맞는 대화를 완성하세요.

> 보기
>
> I don't think I can urinate right now.
> Be sure that the labels on the containers are facing outward.
> You need to urinate in this container and defecate in the other.

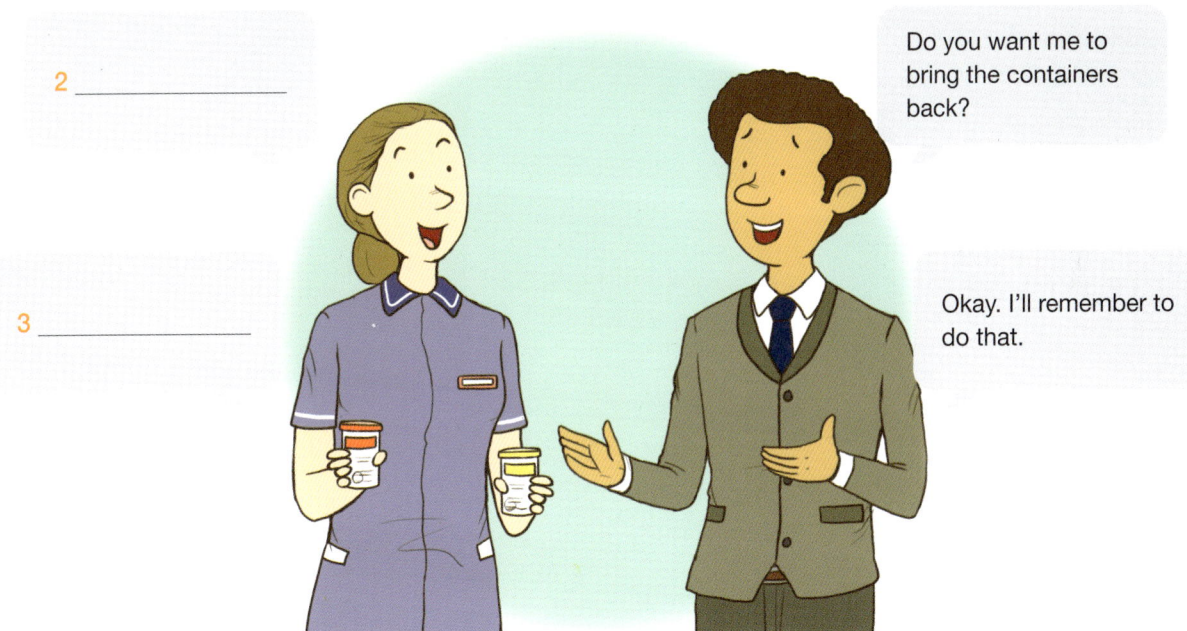

We need both a urine sample and a stool sample from you.

1 _____

2 _____

Do you want me to bring the containers back?

Okay. I'll remember to do that.

3 _____

B 주어진 세 가지 상황을 이용하여, 파트너와 함께 각 상황에 맞는 대화를 연습해 보세요.

Situation	(a)	(b)
1	are going to run	Could you drink some water
2	have to do	Why don't you get some water
3	need to conduct	Can you drink a bit of water

Nurse   Dr. White isn't sure what's wrong with you. So we (a)_____ some tests. We need a urine sample and a stool sample.

Patient   I don't have to urinate right now.

Nurse   That's fine. (b)_____ and wait a few minutes? . . . Okay, Mr. Taylor. Do you think you're ready?

Patient   I'll try now.

Reading & Listening

다음 지문을 읽고, 음성을 들어 보세요.

Nurses' Working Schedules

Track 30

The nurses at most hospitals work two kinds of shifts: 8-hour shifts and 12-hour shifts. For nurses with 8-hour shifts, the day shift usually runs from 7 AM to 3:30 PM, the evening shift runs from 3 PM to 11:30 PM, and the night shift runs from 11 PM to 7:30 AM. For nurses with 12-hour shifts, the day shift runs from 7 AM to 7:30 PM, and the night shift runs from 7 PM to 7:30 AM. These days, many hospitals have a shortage of nurses, so they [1]prefer their nurses to work 12-hour shifts. However, some nurses work shorter shifts. For example, nurses sometimes work 4-hour shifts. Part-time nurses or nurses filling in for absent coworkers usually work these short shifts. Some nurses dislike the 12-hour shifts. They worry about making mistakes when they work long hours. Other nurses do not [2]mind working long shifts.

Words & Phrases

shift a working period　**run** to last for a certain amount of time
shortage a lack of something　**fill in for** to do someone else's work for a short period of time　**mind** to care

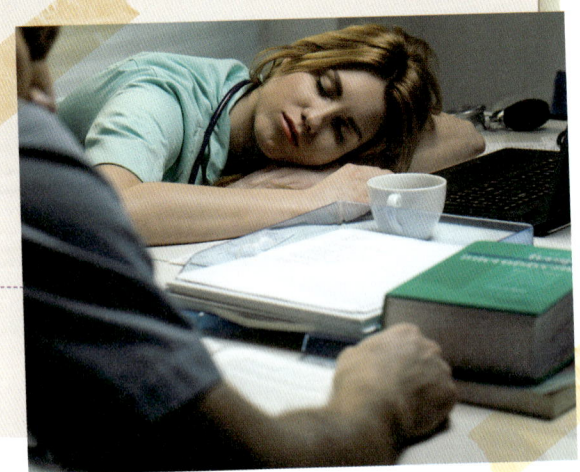

Basic Grammar

① prefer + 목적어 + to V　목적어가 ~하는 것을 선호하다

동사 prefer는 to부정사와 함께 쓰여 '~하는 것을 선호하다'라는 뜻으로 사용된다. 본문에서처럼 prefer와 to부정사 사이에 목적어가 오면 '(주어는) 목적어가 ~하는 것을 선호하다'라는 뜻이 된다.

This hospital prefers the nurses to work 8-hour shifts.　이 병원은 간호사들이 8시간 교대 근무로 일하는 것을 선호한다.
I prefer you to stay inside while you are getting better.　회복하시는 동안에는 안에서만 머무셨으면 좋겠습니다.

② mind -ing　~하는 것을 꺼리다

동사 mind는 '꺼리다'라는 뜻으로, 동명사만을 목적어로 취하는 동사이다.

Some nurses don't mind cleaning vomit.　일부 간호사는 토사물을 치우는 것을 꺼리지 않는다.
Do you mind using a bedpan?　환자용 변기 사용하는 것을 꺼리시나요?

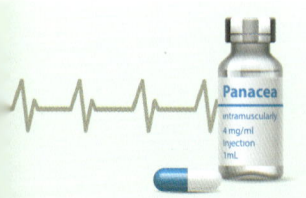

환자만 돌보지 말고 자신도 돌봐 주세요.

간호사는 매우 힘든 직업입니다. 밤이라고 해서 아픈 사람이 없는 것은 아니니, 누군가는 야간 근무를 해야 하지요. 야간 근무를 하다 보면 밤낮이 뒤바뀐 생활에 불면증이 생기기도 쉽습니다. 수면 패턴이 불규칙해지면, 몸이 피곤한 것은 물론이거니와 신경이 곤두서 쉽게 흥분하게 되어 실수하기도 더 쉬워지지요. 간호사라는 직업 특성상 야간 근무에서 완전히 벗어나기는 어려우니, 다른 사람들에 비해 건강 관리에 더 각별히 신경 써야 합니다. 뻔한 말이지만, 건강한 식습관과 적절한 운동, 충분한 스트레스 관리가 그 바탕이 되어야겠지요.

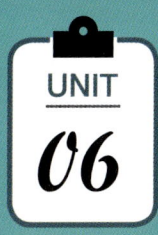

UNIT 06 Examinations II

Warmup

다음은 MRI 검사실에 들어가기 전 환자의 모습입니다. 검사 중 몸에 지닐 수 없는 물건에 모두 체크해 보세요.

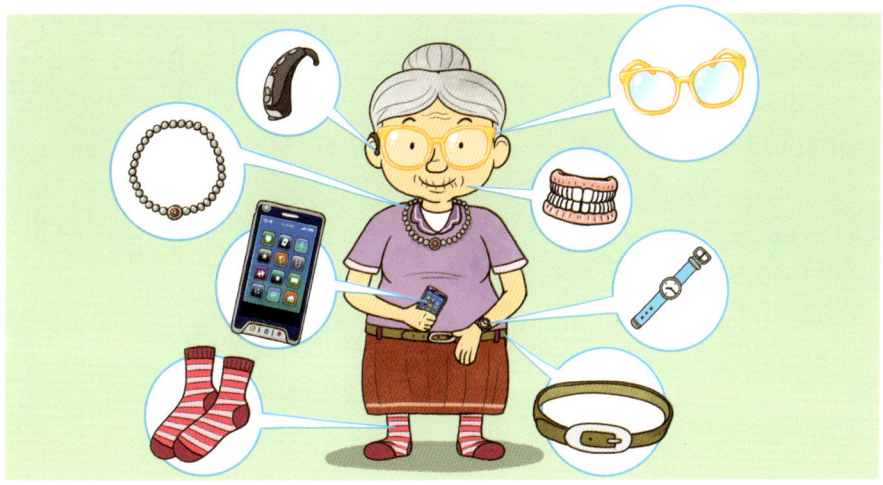

| hearing aid ☐ | glasses ☐ | necklace ☐ | false teeth ☐ |
| cell phone ☐ | watch ☐ | socks ☐ | belt ☐ |

Vocabulary

주어진 의미에 어울리는 단어를 고르세요.

1. remove •   • a. to take off
2. stomach •   • b. unmoving
3. still •   • c. belly
4. swelling •   • d. to move one's hand back and forth on something
5. rub •   • e. the enlargement of a body part; inflammation

Warmup Listening   문장을 듣고 그에 맞는 대답을 고르세요.   Track 31

1. _____
   a. I'm wearing a couple of rings.   b. Both of these are gold rings.
2. _____
   a. Yes, that's my stomach.   b. It's really cold.
3. _____
   a. That's the correct position.   b. Like this?

Unit 06 | 51

Conversation I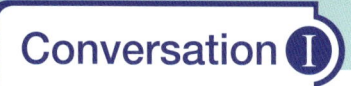

다음 대화를 듣고, 파트너와 함께 대화를 연습해 보세요.

MRI Scans

Track 32

Nurse: We're giving you an MRI exam. ¹Are you wearing any jewelry? And do you have any bank cards or credit cards in your wallet?

Patient: Yes, I have a couple of cards. I'm wearing a necklace, too.

Nurse: ²You need to remove the necklace. You should set your wallet aside as well. You can't have anything metallic in the machine. Now, the process is very simple. Please lie down right here.

Patient: Okay. How do I get in?

Nurse: Just lie on your back. ³You must remain still during the entire process. Please don't move, or else we'll have to do the exam again. You're going to hear some loud noises, but there's nothing to worry about. Everything will be over in a few minutes. Are you ready to begin?

Patient: Yes, I am.

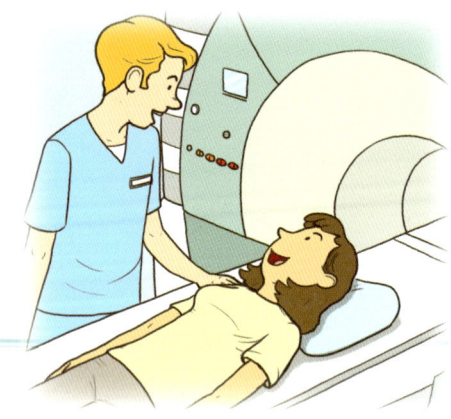

» Key Expressions

❶ Are you wearing any jewelry?   액세서리 착용하고 계신 것 있나요?

MRI 검사 전에 환자가 목걸이, 귀걸이와 같은 액세서리를 착용하고 있는지 확인하는 표현으로, wear뿐만 아니라 have ~ on도 '~을 착용하고 있다'는 뜻으로 사용할 수 있다.

Do you have a watch on you?   시계를 차고 계신가요?

❷ You need to remove the necklace.   목걸이를 빼셔야 합니다.

환자에게 MRI 검사 전에 목걸이를 빼야 한다는 표현이다.

You cannot wear your hearing aid during the test.   검사 중에는 보청기를 착용하실 수 없습니다.
Metal objects are not allowed into the MRI scanning room.   금속 제품은 MRI 촬영실 내에 가지고 들어가실 수 없습니다.

❸ You must remain still during the entire process.   전 과정 동안 가만히 계셔야 합니다.

검사가 진행되는 과정 내내 움직이지 말고 가만히 있어야 한다고 환자에게 당부하는 표현이다. remain 대신 stay나 keep을 사용할 수도 있다.

Please stay [keep] still while you are in the machine.   기계 안에 있는 동안에는 가만히 계세요.
If you move during the scan, we might have to start over.   촬영 중에 움직이시면, 처음부터 다시 시작해야 할 수도 있습니다.

Useful Phrases ➕

눕는 자세를 지시하는 표현

Just lie on your back. 그냥 등을 대고 누우세요.
Lie down on your stomach. 배를 대고 누우세요(엎드리세요).
Please lie face down. 얼굴을 아래로 하고 누우세요(엎드리세요).
Lie on your side and hug your legs. 옆으로 누워서 다리를 안으세요.

Basic Drills

A 주어진 문장에 어울리는 대답을 고르세요.

1. Do you have any bank cards or credit cards in your wallet?
2. Are you ready to begin?
3. How do I get in?

a. Yes, I am.
b. Yes, I have a couple of cards.
c. Just lie on your back.

B 괄호 안의 말을 순서대로 배열하여, 주어진 의미를 영어로 표현하세요.

1. 액세서리 착용하고 계신 것 있나요? (any / you / jewelry / are / wearing)

   _____

2. 목걸이를 빼셔야 합니다. (the necklace / need to / remove / you)

   _____

3. 전 과정 동안 가만히 계셔야 합니다. (during / still / you must / the entire process / remain)

   _____

Buildup Activities

대화를 듣고 빈칸을 채운 후, 주어진 질문에 답하세요.

Track 33

Nurse	You're going to get an (a)_____. Do you have any jewelry on? Are there any credit cards or (b)_____ in your wallet?
Patient	Yes, there are a few cards. And I'm wearing a (c)_____ as well.
Nurse	Please take off the bracelet and leave your wallet here, too. You can't have anything (d)_____ on you when you're in the machine. All right, it's very easy. Just lie down here.
Patient	What (e)_____ should I be in?
Nurse	Lie on your back. And please remain still the entire time. If you move, we'll have to do the exam over. The machine is noisy, but don't worry. This will last about (f)_____. Shall we begin?
Patient	Let's do it.

1. What does the nurse tell the patient to remove?
   a. her ring
   b. her earrings
   c. her bracelet

2. How long will the scan last?
   a. 2 minutes
   b. 10 minutes
   c. 20 minutes

Conversation II

다음 대화를 듣고, 파트너와 함께 대화를 연습해 보세요.

Ultrasound Scans

Nurse: Mr. Sanders, your doctor has ordered an ultrasound scan on you. ¹She wants to know what is causing the swelling in your body. So please lie down on your back on the examination table here.

Patient: All right.

Nurse: Now, just pull your shirt up a bit and be still for a while . . .

Doctor: Hi, Mr. Sanders. I'm Dr. Min. ²I'm going to rub some jelly on your stomach. It's going to feel cold.

Patient: You're right. It is cold. What is this for?

Doctor: It helps the ultrasound work well. It transmits sound waves, so it produces better images. Please don't move as I start using the transducer . . . Okay, ³please turn to your left a bit.

Patient: Like this?

Doctor: Yes, that's perfect . . .

Key Expressions

❶ She wants to know what is causing the swelling in your body.
의사 선생님께서 무엇이 환자분 몸을 붓게 하는지 알고 싶어하십니다.
어떠한 검사를 하기 전에, 환자에게 그 검사를 왜 하는지 알려 주는 표현이다.
We need to find [figure] out why it hurts so badly. 왜 그렇게 심하게 아픈지 알아내야 합니다.

❷ I'm going to rub some jelly on your stomach. 환자분 배에 젤을 조금 발라 드릴 겁니다.
이 표현은 젤, 연고, 로션 등을 발라 주겠다고 할 때 사용할 수 있다. rub 대신 put이나 apply를 사용할 수도 있다.
I will apply some anesthetic cream on your arm. 팔에 마취 연고를 조금 발라 드리겠습니다.
Let me put some cooling salve on your bruises. 멍든 곳에 진정 연고를 조금 발라 드리겠습니다.

❸ Please turn to your left a bit. 왼쪽으로 조금 돌아누워 주세요.
누워 있는 환자에게 다른 자세를 요청하는 말이다.
Please lift your legs higher for me. 다리를 더 높게 들어 주세요.

Useful Phrases

환자의 옷에 대해 요청하는 표현

Pull your shirt up a bit. 셔츠를 조금 올려 주세요.
Lift your shirt up to your chest. 셔츠를 가슴까지 올려 주세요.
Pull down your pants. 바지를 내려 주세요.
Raise your skirt. 치마를 올려 주세요.
Roll up your sleeve for a shot. 주사를 놓게 소매를 걷어 주세요.

Basic Drills

A 주어진 문장에 어울리는 대답을 고르세요.

1. It's going to feel cold. • • a. Like this?
2. What is this for? • • b. You're right. It is cold.
3. Please turn to your left a bit. • • c. It helps the ultrasound work well.

B 괄호 안의 말을 순서대로 배열하여, 주어진 의미를 영어로 표현하세요.

1. 의사 선생님께서 무엇이 환자분 몸을 붓게 하는지 알고 싶어하십니다.
   (in your body / to know / the swelling / she wants / what is causing)
   _____

2. 환자분 배에 젤을 조금 발라 드릴 겁니다. (rub / on / I'm going to / your stomach / some jelly)
   _____

3. 왼쪽으로 조금 돌아누워 주세요. (to / please turn / left / your / a bit)
   _____

Buildup Activities

대화를 듣고 빈칸을 채운 후, 주어진 질문에 답하세요.

Nurse	Mr. Jenkins, the doctor wants to do an (a)_____ scan on you. We need to look at the (b)_____ part of your body. Can you get onto the examination table, please?
Patient	All right.
Nurse	Please (c)_____ your shirt to expose your stomach and wait for a moment . . .
Doctor	I'm going to put some (d)_____ on your stomach. It's pretty cold.
Patient	Yeah, it is. What is the jelly for?
Doctor	It helps (e)_____ sound waves better, so it makes better images. Please don't move while I am using the transducer . . . All right, can you turn to the (f)_____?
Patient	Like this?
Doctor	Yes, exactly.

1. What does the nurse tell the patient to do?
   a. rub some jelly on his stomach
   b. expose part of his stomach
   c. hold the transducer

2. How does the doctor tell the patient to change positions?
   a. by turning to the right
   b. by turning to the left
   c. by lying on his stomach

Job Simulation I

A 〈보기〉에서 적절한 말을 찾아, 각 그림의 상황에 맞는 대화를 완성하세요.

> 보기
> You have to remain still during the entire process.
> You need to remove the earrings and necklace.
> Are you wearing any kind of jewelry?

1 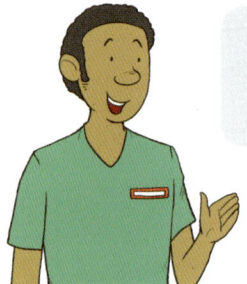 _____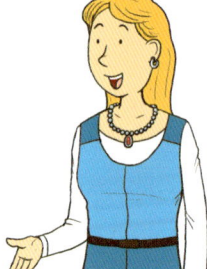
Yes, I'm wearing earrings and a necklace.

2 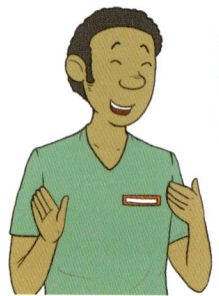 _____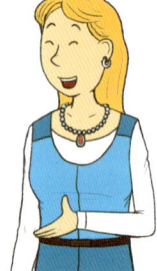
All right. I'll set them down here.

3 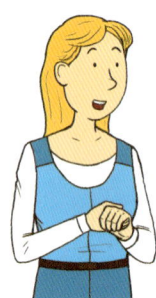 What should I do during the exam?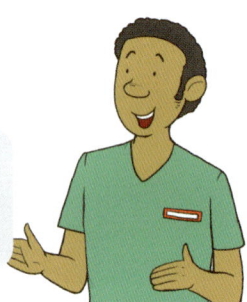
_____

B 주어진 세 가지 상황을 이용하여, 파트너와 함께 각 상황에 맞는 대화를 연습해 보세요.

Situation	(a)	(b)
1	anything made of metal	Please take off
2	jewelry of any type	I want you to remove
3	any jewelry made of metal	You have to remove

Nurse   We're giving you an MRI exam. Are you wearing (a)_____? And do you have any bank cards or credit cards in your wallet?

Patient   Yes, I have a couple of cards. I'm wearing a necklace, too.

Nurse   (b)_____ the necklace. You should set your wallet aside as well. You can't have anything metallic in the machine.

Job Simulation II

A 〈보기〉에서 적절한 말을 찾아, 각 그림의 상황에 맞는 대화를 완성하세요.

> 보기
> I'm going to put some of this jelly on your stomach.
> We have to figure out what is causing the swelling in your body.
> What is this jelly for?

1

Why are you going to do an ultrasound scan on me?

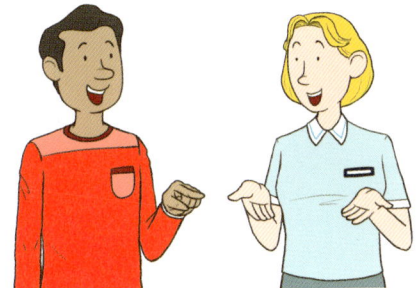

_____

2

_____

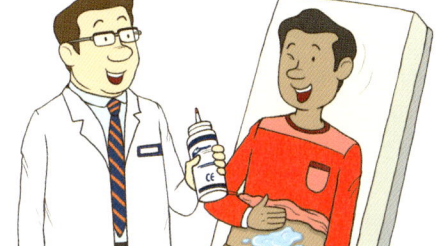

It feels very cold.

3

_____

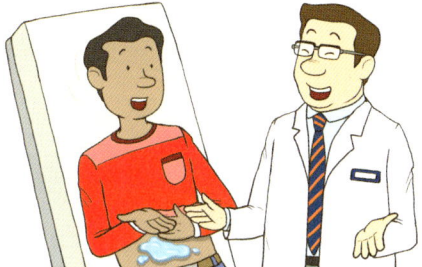

It helps the ultrasound work well, so it produces better images.

B 주어진 세 가지 상황을 이용하여, 파트너와 함께 각 상황에 맞는 대화를 연습해 보세요.

Situation	(a)	(b)	(c)
1	wants to do an ultrasound scan on you	lie down	expose your stomach
2	thinks you need an ultrasound scan	please get up	unbutton your gown
3	believes an ultrasound scan would be good for you	please get up and lie down	pull your shirt up

Nurse   Mr. Sanders, your doctor (a)_____. She wants to know what is causing the swelling in your body. So (b)_____ on the examination table here.

Patient   All right.

Nurse   Now, just (c)_____ and be still for a while . . .

Reading & Listening

다음 지문을 읽고, 음성을 들어 보세요.

The Importance of Teamwork for Nurses

Track 36

Teamwork is integral for nurses. They must work well with other nurses and doctors. When nurses have good teamwork, there are a number of benefits. First, medical care is becoming more complicated and specialized these days. Patients often require the services of several nurses in different departments. These nurses have to work well together to ¹provide the patient with optimal care. In addition, good teamwork reduces the number of mistakes. Since many nurses may assist a single patient, they need to work well as a team to be sure the patient gets the proper medical care, medication, and other attention he or she needs. Finally, patients and their families need to see the nurses working well with one another and with doctors. This gives the patients and their families more confidence in the hospital staff and makes their visits to the hospital much ²more comfortable.

Words & Phrases

teamwork the ability to work well with others **integral** very important
complicated difficult; complex **optimal** the best **proper** correct; good; effective

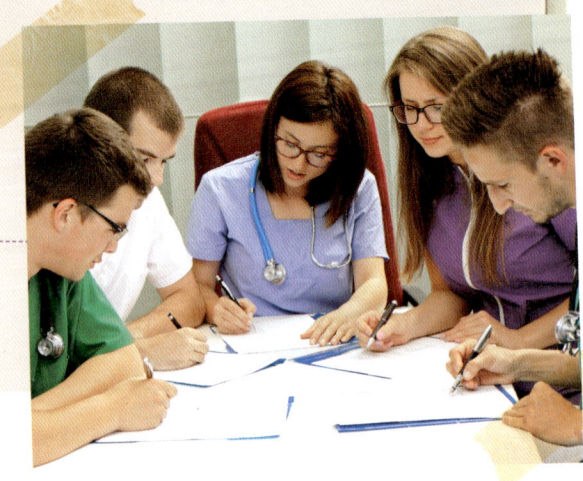

Basic Grammar

① provide A with B A에게 B를 제공하다

동사 provide는 '제공하다'라는 뜻으로, 전치사 with와 함께 provide A with B(A에게 B를 제공하다)라는 형식으로 쓰일 수 있다. 전치사 with 대신 for가 쓰이는 경우, A와 B의 자리가 바뀐다.

We provide every new mom with basic supplies, such as a can of powdered formula and a pack of diapers.
저희는 모든 산모에게 가루 분유 한 캔과 기저귀 한 팩 같은 기본 용품을 제공합니다.
Some hospitals provide childcare service for their visitors. 일부 병원은 방문객에게 탁아 서비스를 제공한다.

② 형용사의 비교급

일반적으로 형용사의 비교급은 형용사 뒤에 -er을 붙여서 나타내지만, 본문의 comfortable처럼 음절이 긴 형용사의 경우 형용사 앞에 more를 붙여서 비교급을 만든다. 참고로 형용사의 비교급 앞에, 본문에 쓰인 much 또는 still, even, far, a lot 같은 부사를 넣으면 '훨씬' 이라는 강조의 의미를 더할 수 있다.

This type of cancer is far more curable. 이런 종류의 암은 치료될 가능성이 훨씬 더 크다.

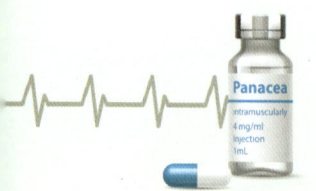

초음파 검사의 원리가 궁금해요!

초음파 검사를 앞두고 들뜬 마음으로 병원을 찾는 임신부가 많습니다. 뱃속에 있는 아기를 볼 수 있다는 생각에 설레는 것이지요. 병원의 초음파 검사는 돌고래나 박쥐가 사용하는 초음파와 그 원리가 비슷합니다. 예를 들어, 박쥐가 초음파를 발사하면 장애물 등에 부딪혀 반사된 초음파가 박쥐 귀에 되돌아와서 장애물을 피할 수 있는데요. 초음파 검사도 마찬가지입니다. 초음파 기계가 인체의 뼈나 조직에 초음파를 보내면, 초음파가 반사되어 되돌아옵니다. 그러면 기계가 이 반사된 초음파를 이미지로 바꾸는 것이지요. 이러한 초음파 기술 덕에 뱃속의 태아뿐만 아니라 간, 신장, 유방, 갑상선 등도 간편하게 검사할 수 있게 되었습니다.

UNIT 07 Giving Orientation about Hospitalization

Warmup
다음은 병실 내부의 모습입니다. 각 시설에 해당하는 단어를 아래에서 찾아 써 보세요.

1. _____
2. _____
3. _____
4. _____
5. _____
6. _____
7. _____
8. _____

| bedsheet | television | chair | bedside table | cabinet | folding table | window | pillow |

Vocabulary
주어진 의미에 어울리는 단어를 고르세요.

1. press •   • a. a cushion used to rest one's head on
2. nap •   • b. items used to clean oneself such as soap or shampoo
3. pillow •   • c. normal; usual
4. regular •   • d. to push
5. toiletries •   • e. a short sleep in the morning or afternoon

Track 37

Warmup Listening
문장을 듣고 그에 맞는 대답을 고르세요.

1. _____
   a. When you need something, press it.   b. What did you press the button for?

2. _____
   a. You can visit him soon.   b. They are from 9 AM to 8 PM.

3. _____
   a. Let me talk to the dietician.   b. Yes, you're drinking regular milk now.

Conversation I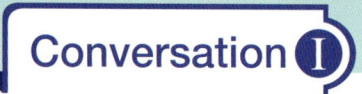

다음 대화를 듣고, 파트너와 함께 대화를 연습해 보세요.

Describing Patients' Rooms

Nurse	This is your room, Mr. Hamilton. You'll stay here until you go home. Here are your bed and bedside table.
Patient	What's this button for?
Nurse	It's the call button. ¹When you need help, just press the button. A nurse will come to see you immediately.
Patient	Should I use it if I need some pain medicine?
Nurse	Yes, that's right. You're going to get three meals a day. ²We serve breakfast at 8 AM and lunch at noon. You'll get your dinner at 6 PM.
Patient	What about visiting hours? My wife and children are planning to visit me every day.
Nurse	³The hospital's visiting hours are 10 AM to 8 PM on weekdays and 9 AM to 10 PM on weekends.
Patient	Thank you for explaining everything.

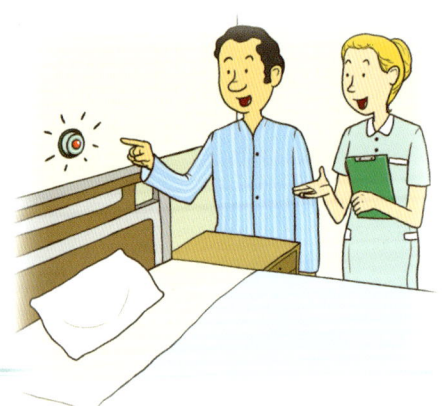

Key Expressions

❶ **When you need help, just press the button.** 도움이 필요하실 때, 버튼만 눌러 주세요.
입원 환자에게 도움이 필요하면 호출 버튼을 눌러 간호사를 불러 달라는 표현이다.

Let us know if you need anything by pressing this button. 무엇이든 필요하시면 이 버튼을 눌러 저희에게 알려 주세요.
If you push the button, a nurse will come in right away. 버튼을 누르시면, 간호사가 바로 올 겁니다.

❷ **We serve breakfast at 8 AM and lunch at noon.** 아침은 오전 8시에, 점심은 정오에 제공합니다.
입원 환자에게 병원의 식사 시간을 안내하는 표현이다. 특정 시각 앞에는 전치사 at이 온다.

❸ **The hospital's visiting hours are 10 AM to 8 PM on weekdays and 9 AM to 10 PM on weekends.**
병원의 면회 시간은 평일에는 오전 10시부터 오후 8시까지고, 주말에는 오전 9시부터 오후 10시까지입니다.
면회 시간을 안내하는 표현이다. on weekdays(평일에)나 on weekends(주말에)와 같이 요일 앞에는 전치사 on이 온다.

Your family can visit you between 9 AM and 8 PM every day. 가족분들은 매일 오전 9시에서 오후 8시 사이에 환자분을 방문하실 수 있습니다.

Useful Phrases ➕

병실에 있는 물품을 소개하는 표현

This is the call button. 이것은 호출 버튼입니다.
You have the bed control here. 여기에 침대 조종 장치가 있습니다.
This is your hospital gown. 이것은 환자복입니다.
You can use this bedpan. 이 환자용 변기를 사용하시면 됩니다.

Basic Drills

A 주어진 문장에 어울리는 대답을 고르세요.

1. What's this button for? • • a. The hospital's visiting hours are 10 AM to 8 PM on weekdays and 9 AM to 10 PM on weekends.

2. Should I use it if I need some pain medicine? • • b. Yes, that's right.

3. What about visiting hours? • • c. It's the call button.

B 괄호 안의 말을 순서대로 배열하여, 주어진 의미를 영어로 표현하세요.

1. 도움이 필요하실 때, 버튼만 눌러 주세요. (the button / when / help / just press / you need)

   _____

2. 아침은 오전 8시에, 점심은 정오에 제공합니다. (breakfast / we serve / lunch / at noon / at 8 AM / and)

   _____

3. 병원의 면회 시간은 평일에는 오전 10시부터 오후 8시까지고, 주말에는 오전 9시부터 오후 10시까지입니다.
   (9 AM to 10 PM / are / 10 AM to 8 PM / and / the hospital's visiting hours / on weekends / on weekdays)

   _____

Buildup Activities

대화를 듣고 빈칸을 채운 후, 주어진 질문에 답하세요.   Track 39

Nurse	Here is your room, Mr. Emerson. You'll stay here until you (a)_____. There are your bed and bedside table.
Patient	What's (b)_____?
Nurse	It's the call button. Press that button if you need to see (c)_____. One of us will come here at once.
Patient	If I am (d)_____, should I press it?
Nurse	Yes, you should. In addition, you'll eat three times each day. We serve breakfast at 7:30 and lunch at noon. Your dinner will arrive at 6:30.
Patient	What are the hospital's (e)_____? My family is planning to visit me each day.
Nurse	(f)_____, visiting hours run from 9 AM to 7 PM, and they last from 8 AM to 9 PM on weekends.
Patient	Thanks for your explanations.

1. When should the patient press the button?

   a. when he is sleepy

   b. when he is in pain

   c. when he is hungry

2. When do the hospital's visiting hours end on weekdays?

   a. at 7 PM   b. at 8 PM   c. at 9 PM

Conversation II

다음 대화를 듣고, 파트너와 함께 대화를 연습해 보세요.

Answering Patients' Questions about Hospital Life

Track 40

Patient Excuse me, nurse, but I have a question. My husband would like to take a nap. Can I get a blanket and a pillow for him, please?
Nurse ¹I'm very sorry, but we only provide those to patients. We don't give them to visitors.
Patient I understand. By the way, I have a question about the food here.
Nurse Sure. What is it?
Patient ²Can I get soy milk instead of regular milk? I don't like the taste of regular milk.
Nurse ³I'll talk to the dietician and see if that is okay. Do you have any other questions?
Patient I have one more question. Where can I get toiletries such as a toothbrush and toothpaste?
Nurse There's a convenience store on the basement floor.

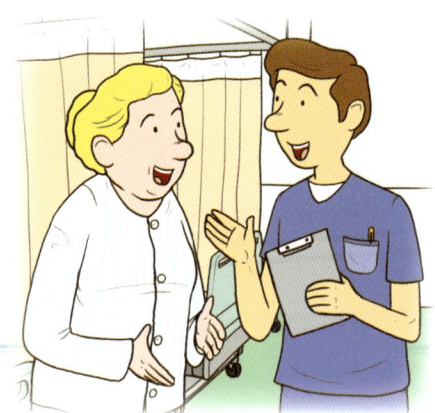

» Key Expressions

❶ I'm very sorry, but we only provide those to patients.   정말 죄송하지만, 그것들은 환자분들에게만 제공합니다.

담요나 베개 등의 물품이 환자에게만 제공된다고 안내하는 표현이다.

I am afraid we are not allowed to give this to visitors.   죄송합니다만, 이것은 방문객에게는 제공할 수 없습니다.
These are for patients only.   이것들은 환자 전용입니다.

❷ Can I get soy milk instead of regular milk?   일반 우유 대신에 두유를 받을 수 있나요?

환자가 일반 우유 대신에 두유를 받을 수 있는지 묻는 표현이다. A instead of B는 'B 대신에 A'라는 의미를 나타낼 때 사용할 수 있다.

Can I come in on Thursday instead of Friday?   금요일 대신 목요일에 방문해도 될까요?
Can I have my lunch later? I'm not feeling hungry right now.   점심을 이따가 먹어도 될까요? 지금은 배가 안 고파서요.

❸ I'll talk to the dietician and see if that is okay.   제가 영양사님에게 이야기해서 그래도 되는지 확인해 보겠습니다.

환자가 요청한 사항이 가능한지 알아보겠다는 표현이다.

Let me check with the doctor about it first.   그것에 대해 먼저 의사 선생님과 상의해 보겠습니다.
Let me see what I can do for you.   제가 무엇을 해 드릴 수 있는지 확인해 보겠습니다.

Useful Phrases

| 더 궁금한 점 있으세요? |

Do you have any other questions?
Are there any other questions?
Is there anything else you would like to know [ask]?
Is there anything else you need?

Basic Drills

A 주어진 문장에 어울리는 대답을 고르세요.

1. Do you have any other questions? • • a. I'm very sorry, but we only provide those to patients.
2. Can I get a blanket and a pillow for him, please? • • b. I have one more question.
3. Can I get soy milk instead of regular milk? • • c. I'll talk to the dietician and see if that is okay.

B 괄호 안의 말을 순서대로 배열하여, 주어진 의미를 영어로 표현하세요.

1. 정말 죄송하지만, 그것들은 환자분들에게만 제공합니다. (but / to patients / I'm very sorry / those / we only provide)
   _____

2. 일반 우유 대신에 두유를 받을 수 있나요? (get / regular milk / soy milk / can I / instead of)
   _____

3. 제가 영양사님에게 이야기해서 그래도 되는지 확인해 보겠습니다. (the dietician / I'll talk / and / see if / to / that is okay)
   _____

Buildup Activities

대화를 듣고 빈칸을 채운 후, 주어진 질문에 답하세요.

Patient	Pardon me, nurse, but I have a question. (a)_____ wants to take a nap. Can you get a blanket and a pillow for him, please?
Nurse	I'm terribly sorry, but we (b)_____ those to patients. We can't let visitors have them.
Patient	That's fine. By the way, I have a question about my food.
Nurse	Sure. What is it?
Patient	Can I get (c)_____ instead of tofu? I don't really like tofu.
Nurse	Let me talk to the (d)_____ and see if that is okay. Are there any other questions?
Patient	Yes, I have one last question. Where can I get toiletries such as (e)_____ and shampoo?
Nurse	There's a (f)_____ on the first floor.

1. Who does the patient want to get a blanket and a pillow for?
   a. her son   b. her husband   c. her brother

2. What food does the patient want to eat?
   a. tofu   b. eggs   c. yogurt

Job Simulation I

A 〈보기〉에서 적절한 말을 찾아, 각 그림의 상황에 맞는 대화를 완성하세요.

> 보기
> When you need assistance, just press it.
> They last from 10 to 7 on weekdays and run from 9 to 8 on weekends.
> We serve breakfast at 8:30 and lunch at noon every day.

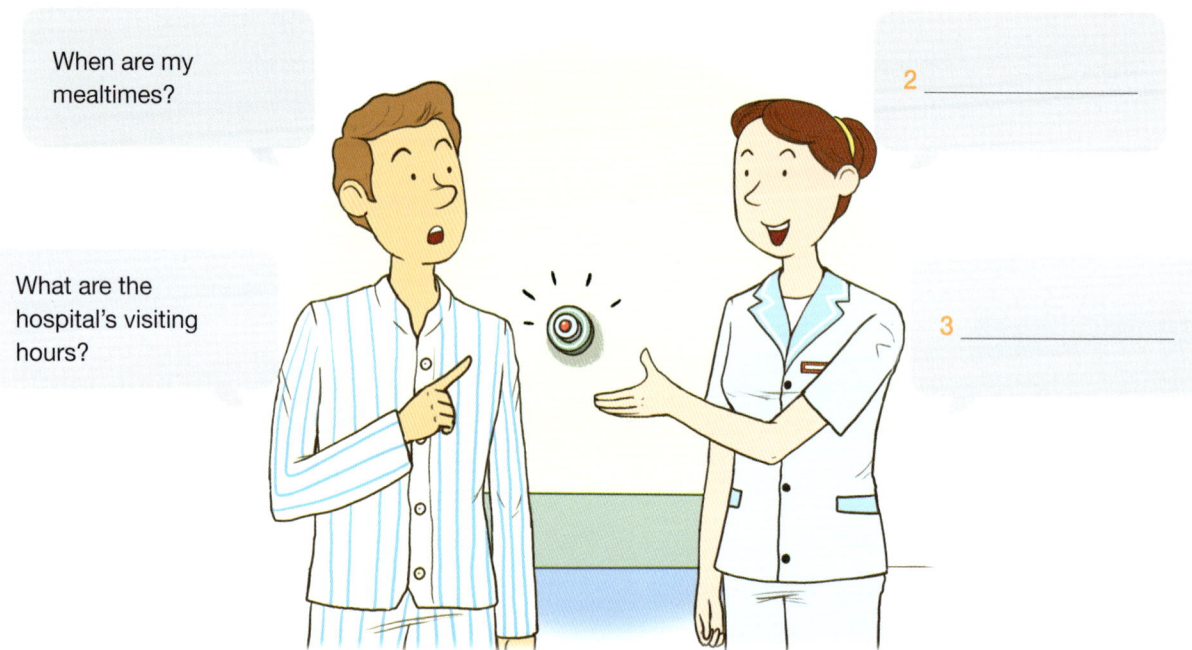

What is the purpose of this button?

1 _____

When are my mealtimes?

2 _____

What are the hospital's visiting hours?

3 _____

B 주어진 세 가지 상황을 이용하여, 파트너와 함께 각 상황에 맞는 대화를 연습해 보세요.

Situation	(a)	(b)
1	around 6:30 PM	What are the visiting hours here
2	at 7:00 in the evening	When are the hospital's visiting hours
3	at approximately 6:15	When are visitors allowed to come

Nurse　We serve breakfast at 8 AM and lunch at noon. You'll get your dinner (a)_____.

Patient　(b)_____? My wife and children are planning to visit me every day.

Nurse　The hospital's visiting hours are 10 AM to 8 PM on weekdays and 9 AM to 10 PM on weekends.

Patient　Thank you for explaining everything.

Job Simulation II

A 〈보기〉에서 적절한 말을 찾아, 각 그림의 상황에 맞는 대화를 완성하세요.

> 보기
> I'll speak to the dietician to see if that is possible.
> I'm sorry, but we only let patients use them.
> May I have soy milk instead of regular milk?

1. Can I get a blanket and a pillow for my husband, please?

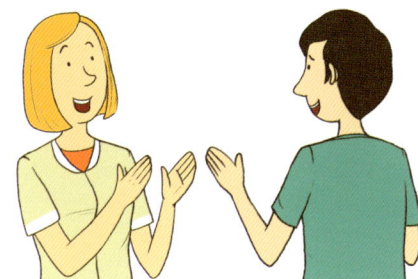

_____

2. What is your question about the food?

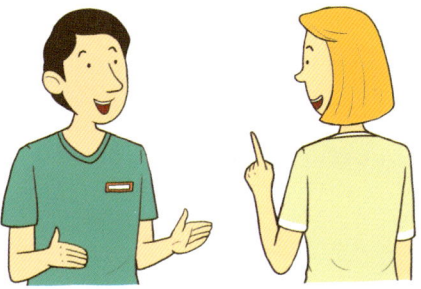

_____

3. I'm a vegan, so I don't eat dairy products.

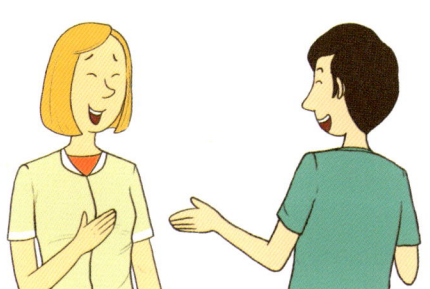

_____

B 주어진 세 가지 상황을 이용하여, 파트너와 함께 각 상황에 맞는 대화를 연습해 보세요.

Situation	(a)	(b)	(c)
1	how regular milk tastes	check with her	some drinks
2	regular milk at all	see if he minds	some snack food for my children
3	the way that regular milk tastes	see if you're allowed to drink it	a few necessities such as soap and shampoo

Patient   Can I get soy milk instead of regular milk? I don't like (a)_____.

Nurse   I'll talk to the dietician and (b)_____.

Patient   I have one more question. Where can I get (c)_____?

Nurse   There's a convenience store on the basement floor.

Reading & Listening
다음 지문을 읽고, 음성을 들어 보세요.

How Nurses Can Cope with Stress

Track 42

[1]Being a nurse can be stressful. Nurses have many patients, so they are constantly busy. In addition, their patients sometimes pass away, which can cause additional stress. Fortunately, there are ways to cope with stress on the job. Nurses should have good communication with their coworkers and patients, and they should be as organized as possible. Those two things will make their jobs easier. They also need a mentor or someone they can talk with when they have problems. [2]By speaking about their problems, they can get advice on handling them. Nurses should also keep themselves in good shape. They can do that by exercising regularly and eating healthy food. They should have hobbies, too. Hobbies will help them keep their minds off their jobs when they aren't working. Finally, nurses should take some time off if their lives ever become too stressful because of their jobs.

Words & Phrases
pass away to die **additional** extra; more than normal **cope with** to handle; to deal with **mentor** an older, experienced person who provides advice or assistance to another person **take time off** to take vacation; to stop working for some time

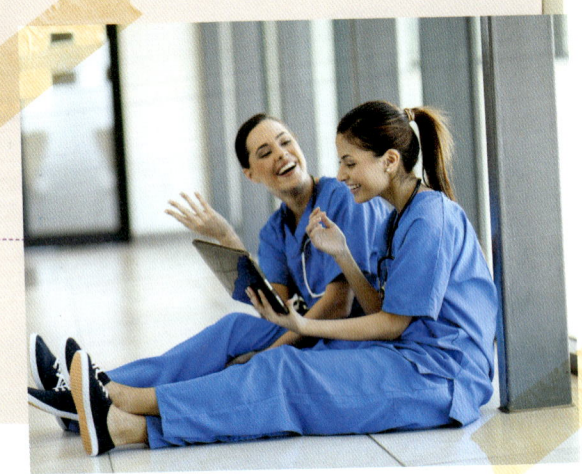

» Basic Grammar

❶ 동명사

동명사(-ing)는 '~하는 것'이라는 뜻으로, 동사의 성질을 지니고 있으면서 명사의 역할을 한다. 본문의 Being a nurse는 '간호사인 것'이라는 뜻으로, 명사로서 주어 자리에 사용되었다.

Working the night shift can be difficult.   야간 근무로 일하는 것은 힘들 수 있다.
Taking care of patients is very rewarding.   환자들을 돌보는 것은 매우 보람 있다.

❷ by -ing ~함으로써

'~에 의하여'라는 뜻의 전치사 by와 동명사(-ing)가 짝을 이루어, '~하는 것에 의하여', 즉 '~함으로써'라는 의미를 나타낸다.

By pressing this button, you can call a nurse.   이 버튼을 누름으로써, 간호사를 부르실 수 있습니다.
You can get to room 322 by taking the elevator over there.   저쪽에 있는 엘리베이터를 타고 322호실에 가실 수 있습니다.

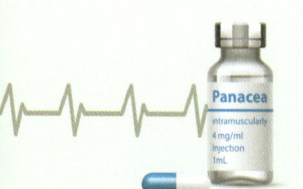

TIPS&TIPS

극한 직업, 응급 간호사

응급 간호사는 응급 환자를 돌보는 등록 간호사(RN)를 말합니다. 응급 상황은 환자에게뿐만 아니라 응급 간호사에게도 몹시 위험한데요. 첫째로, 환자가 폭력적으로 돌변해 간호사를 공격하는 경우가 있습니다. 둘째로, 감염병에 걸린 환자를 돌보다 병이 옮기도 합니다. 아프리카에서는 에볼라 바이러스에 감염된 환자들을 치료하던 간호사들이 에볼라에 감염되기도 했지요. 그뿐인가요? 응급실에는 위험한 화학물질이나 날카로운 물건이 많기 때문에, 근무하다 다칠 수도 있습니다. 그 밖에도 덩치 큰 환자를 옮기다가 다치거나, 지나친 스트레스와 피로로 건강을 해치는 경우도 있다고 하니, 응급 간호사는 정말 극한 직업이네요.

UNIT 08 Taking Care of Patients

Warmup

다음 사진들을 드레싱을 교체하는 순서에 맞게 배열해 보세요.

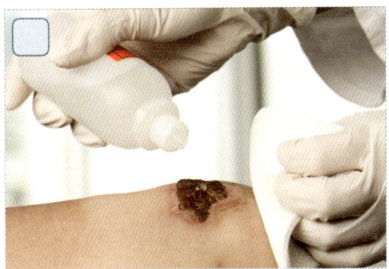
disinfect a cut

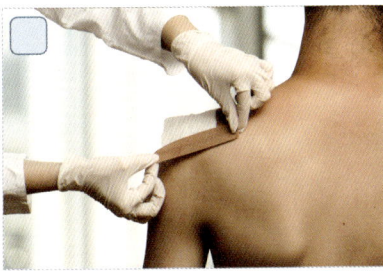
put on a sterile dressing

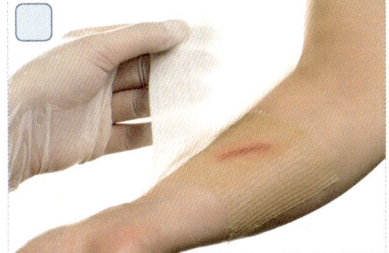
remove an old dressing

Vocabulary

주어진 의미에 어울리는 단어를 고르세요.

1. dressing
2. position
3. sterile
4. itch
5. infected

a. a bandage
b. very clean; having no germs
c. to have a feeling that makes one want to scratch
d. the way a person is sitting or lying down
e. having a disease or germs

Warmup Listening

Track 43

문장을 듣고 그에 맞는 대답을 고르세요.

1.
   a. Yes, that's how I feel.
   b. I feel much better today.
2.
   a. You should stop scratching.
   b. Then I can replace the dressing.
3.
   a. Lying in the same position can cause bedsores.
   b. You are still lying in bed.

Conversation I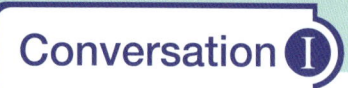

다음 대화를 듣고, 파트너와 함께 대화를 연습해 보세요.

Changing Patients' Dressings

Nurse	Good morning, Mr. Hampton. How do you feel today?
Patient	I think I'm getting better. ¹I feel better today than I did yesterday.
Nurse	I'm glad to hear that. I have to change your dressing now.
Patient	Thank you. ²It is really starting to itch a lot.
Nurse	Why don't you lie back on the bed? Then, I can replace the dressing with a new sterile one. That will help stop the itching.
Patient	Sure.
Nurse	Hmm . . . Your cut is healing well, and it's not infected at all. ³You appear to be improving rapidly.
Patient	That's great news. Thanks.

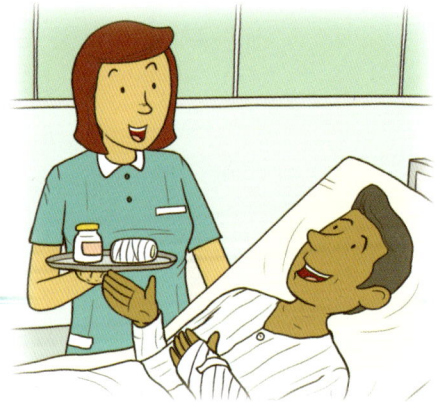

» Key Expressions

❶ I feel better today than I did yesterday.   오늘은 어제보다 몸 상태가 좋아요.

몸 상태나 기분이 어제보다 좋다고 나타내는 표현이다.

My arm is feeling much stronger than it was last week.   지난주보다 팔에 훨씬 더 힘이 들어가는 것 같아요.

❷ It is really starting to itch a lot.   정말 많이 가려워지기 시작했어요.

붕대를 감은 부위 등이 가려워지기 시작했다는 표현이다.

It is really itchy. = It really itches.   정말 가려워요.
It's so itchy that I want to pick at my dressing.   너무 가려워서 붕대를 긁고 싶어요.

❸ You appear to be improving rapidly.   빠르게 회복하고 계신 것 같습니다.

이 표현은 환자가 빠르게 회복하고 있는 것 같다고 말할 때 사용할 수 있다. improve 대신에 recover나 get better도 사용할 수 있다.

It looks like you are recovering well.   잘 회복하고 계신 것 같습니다.
You sure are getting better.   확실히 회복하고 계십니다.

Useful Phrases ➕

좋은 소식이네요. [그거 잘됐네요.]

= That's great news.
= I'm glad to hear that.
= What good news!
= That's good to hear.

Basic Drills

A 주어진 문장에 어울리는 대답을 고르세요.

1. I have to change your dressing now. •   • a. Thank you.
2. How do you feel today? •   • b. That's great news.
3. You appear to be improving rapidly. •   • c. I feel better today than I did yesterday.

B 괄호 안의 말을 순서대로 배열하여, 주어진 의미를 영어로 표현하세요.

1. 오늘은 어제보다 몸 상태가 좋아요. (I did / better today / I feel / yesterday / than)

   _____

2. 정말 많이 가려워지기 시작했어요. (starting / a lot / it is / really / to itch)

   _____

3. 빠르게 회복하고 계신 것 같습니다. (rapidly / you / be improving / appear / to)

   _____

Buildup Activities

대화를 듣고 빈칸을 채운 후, 주어진 질문에 답하세요.

Track **45**

Nurse	Good morning, Mr. Pennington. How are you doing this morning?
Patient	I think I'm improving. I feel (a)_____ better today than I did yesterday.
Nurse	That's great news. It's time for me to change your (b)_____.
Patient	Good. It (c)_____ a lot.
Nurse	Would you please lie down on the bed? Then, I can put a (d)_____ on. That will make you stop itching.
Patient	Okay.
Nurse	Hmm . . . Your cut is (e)_____, but it's not infected. You should start to (f)_____ in a few days.
Patient	That's nice to know. Thank you.

1. How does the patient feel?

   a. much better than yesterday

   b. worse than yesterday

   c. a bit better than yesterday

2. What does the nurse NOT say about the cut?

   a. It is bleeding.

   b. It is not infected.

   c. It is slowly improving.

Conversation II

다음 대화를 듣고, 파트너와 함께 대화를 연습해 보세요.

Telling Patients to Change Positions

Track 46

Nurse	Mr. Thompson, it's four o'clock. You need to change positions.
Patient	Didn't I just do that a while ago?
Nurse	Yes, you did. ¹You ought to change your position every two hours when you are in bed.
Patient	Really? Why do I have to do that?
Nurse	²If you lie in the same position, it will decrease the blood flow to some parts of your body. That will make the tissue there become weaker.
Patient	Is that bad?
Nurse	Yes, it is. ³You can develop bedsores. If those get infected, you'll have some serious problems. That's why we make patients rotate their positions.
Patient	I understand. I'll turn around frequently from now on.

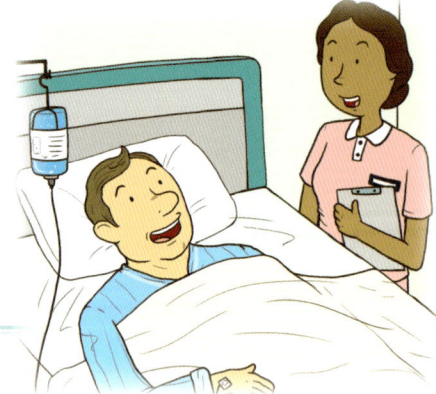

» Key Expressions

❶ You ought to change your position every two hours when you are in bed.

침대에 누워 계실 때는 두 시간마다 자세를 바꾸셔야 합니다.

침대에 장시간 누워 있어야 하는 환자에게 두 시간마다 자세를 바꿔야 한다고 말하고 있다. every 뒤에 시간을 넣으면 '~마다'라는 의미를 나타낼 수 있다.

You should take these pills every 6 hours.   이 알약들을 6시간마다 드셔야 합니다.

❷ If you lie in the same position, it will decrease the blood flow to some parts of your body.

같은 자세로 누워 계시면, 신체 일부로 가는 혈류량이 줄어듭니다.

환자에게 같은 자세로만 누워 있으면 어떻게 되는지 경고하는 표현이다. 이처럼 특정한 행동을 했을 때 어떤 일이 생기는지 환자에게 알려줄 때는 if를 사용할 수 있다.

If you exercise too hard, your back pain will get worse.   운동을 너무 무리하게 하면, 허리 통증이 더 심해질 겁니다.

❸ You can develop bedsores.   욕창이 생길 수 있습니다.

환자에게 욕창이 생길 수 있다고 말할 때 사용한다. 동사 develop 대신 get이나 have도 사용할 수 있다.

There is a chance that you will get bedsores.   욕창이 생길 가능성이 있습니다.

Useful Phrases ➕

누워 있는 환자에게 자세를 바꾸라고 요청하는 표현

You need to change positions. 자세를 바꾸셔야 합니다.
It's time to change positions. 자세를 바꾸실 시간입니다.
Let's change to a new position. 새로운 자세로 바꾸어 봅시다.
Please roll over on your left [right] side. 왼쪽[오른쪽]으로 돌아누워 주세요.

Basic Drills

A 주어진 문장에 어울리는 대답을 고르세요.

1. You need to change positions.
2. Why do I have to do that?
3. That's why we make patients rotate their positions.

a. If you lie in the same position, it will decrease the blood flow to some parts of your body.
b. Didn't I just do that a while ago?
c. I understand.

B 괄호 안의 말을 순서대로 배열하여, 주어진 의미를 영어로 표현하세요.

1. 침대에 누워 계실 때는 두 시간마다 자세를 바꾸셔야 합니다.
   (every / you ought to / you are in bed / two hours / change your position / when)

   _____

2. 같은 자세로 누워 계시면, 신체 일부로 가는 혈류량이 줄어듭니다.
   (the blood flow / in the same position / of your body / it will decrease / if you lie / to some parts)

   _____

3. 욕창이 생길 수 있습니다. (develop / can / you / bedsores)

   _____

Buildup Activities

대화를 듣고 빈칸을 채운 후, 주어진 질문에 답하세요.

Track 47

Nurse   Mr. Kimball, it's five o'clock. It's time to change (a)_____.

Patient Didn't I do that a few hours ago?

Nurse   Yes, you did. But you're supposed to change positions every (b)_____ when you are in bed.

Patient Really? (c)_____ am I supposed to do that?

Nurse   Lying in the same position will (d)_____ the blood flowing to certain parts of your body. That will weaken the tissue in those places.

Patient Is that a bad thing?

Nurse   Yes, it is. You might get (e)_____. Infected bedsores can cause serious problems. That's why patients need to rotate positions regularly.

Patient I understand. I'll be sure to turn (f)_____ in that case.

1. What does the nurse tell the patient to do?
   a. get out of his bed
   b. change his position
   c. get some food

2. What does the patient say he will do?
   a. lie in bed all day
   b. get up and walk around
   c. turn every two hours

Unit 08 | 71

Job Simulation I

Ⓐ 〈보기〉에서 적절한 말을 찾아, 각 그림의 상황에 맞는 대화를 완성하세요.

> 보기
> There is no sign of infection around your cut.
> Excellent. It itches a lot.
> I feel a great deal better today.

How do you feel right now?

1. _____

I need to change your bandage.

2. _____

3. _____

That's excellent news.

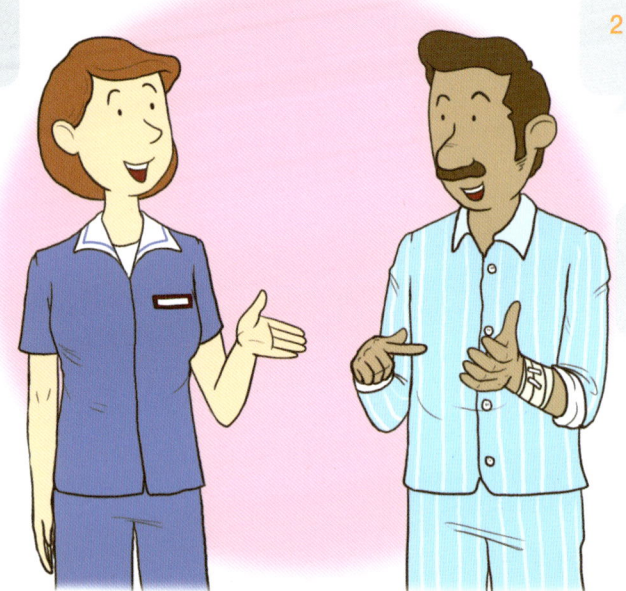

Ⓑ 주어진 세 가지 상황을 이용하여, 파트너와 함께 각 상황에 맞는 대화를 연습해 보세요.

Situation	(a)	(b)
1	make you stop itching	is getting better
2	make the itching go away	looks very good
3	get rid of the itching	seems to be healing well

Nurse   I can replace the dressing with a new sterile one. That will help (a)_____.

Patient   Sure.

Nurse   Hmm . . . Your cut (b)_____, and it's not infected at all. You appear to be improving rapidly.

Patient   That's great news. Thanks.

72 | Taking Care of Patients

Job Simulation II

A 〈보기〉에서 적절한 말을 찾아, 각 그림의 상황에 맞는 대화를 완성하세요.

> 보기
> You need to change positions every two hours when you are in bed.
> Okay. I'll be sure to rotate more often then.
> Lying in the same position will decrease the blood flow to certain parts of your body.

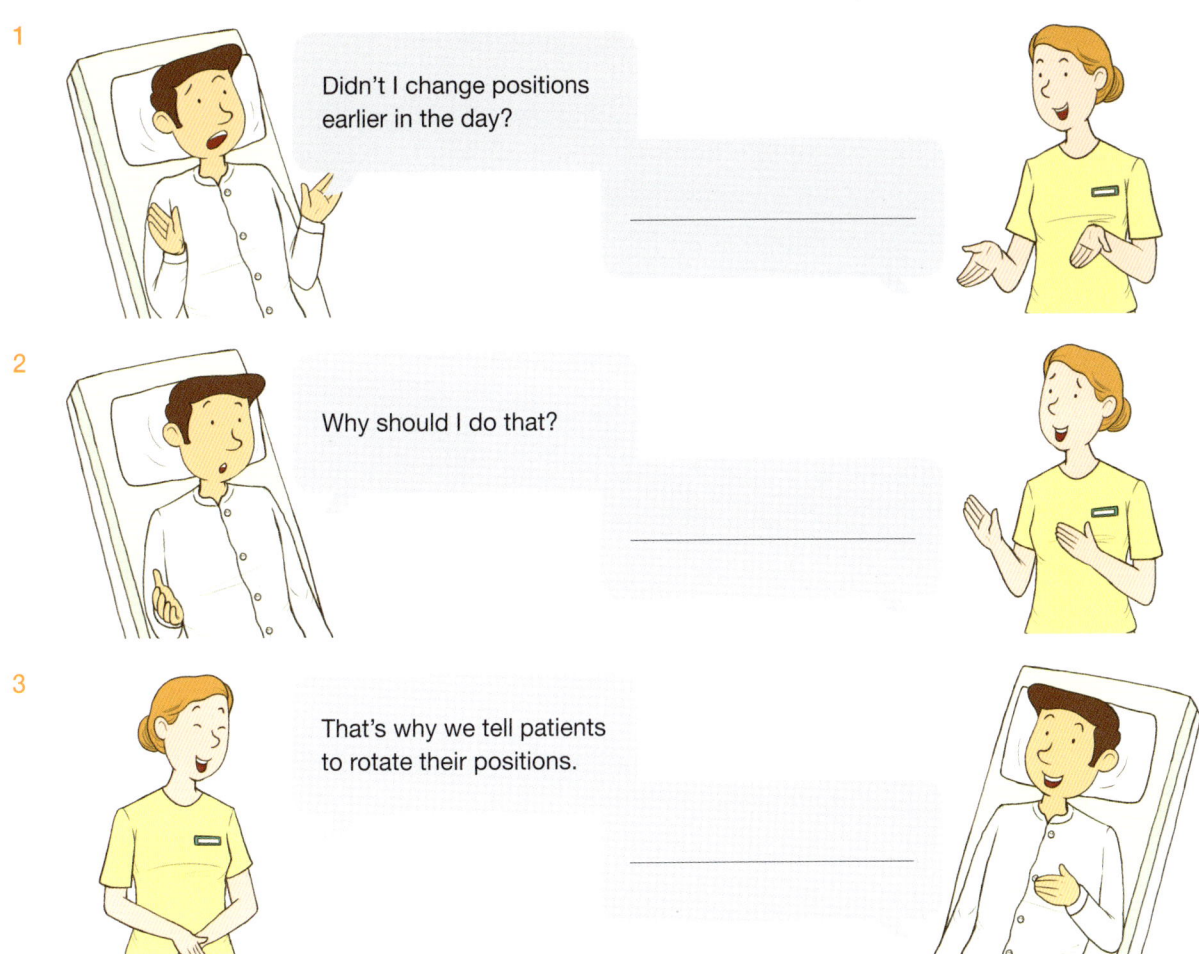

B 주어진 세 가지 상황을 이용하여, 파트너와 함께 각 상황에 맞는 대화를 연습해 보세요.

Situation	(a)	(b)
1	cause less blood to flow	might get bedsores
2	reduce the amount of blood flowing	could develop bedsores
3	make less blood flow	may get some bedsores

Nurse   If you lie in the same position, it will (a)_____ to some parts of your body. That will make the tissue there become weaker.

Patient   Is that bad?

Nurse   Yes, it is. You (b)_____. That's why we make patients rotate their positions.

Patient   I understand. I'll turn around frequently from now on.

Reading & Listening

다음 지문을 읽고, 음성을 들어 보세요.

Fall Prevention Programs

Track 48

According to statistics, around 20% of all inpatients fall down during their stays in hospitals. Around half suffer some kind of injury. Therefore, hospitals do their best to [1]prevent patients from falling. After all, they want their patients to get better, not worse. Many hospitals have fall prevention programs. [2]For instance, the elderly tend to fall down in the bathroom. So hospitals may assign a nurse to assist elderly patients in the bathroom. Nurses also monitor patients' medicine to make sure that it doesn't affect their physical abilities too badly. Hospitals provide alarms for patients to press if they are in danger of falling or have fallen down. Nurses can also use restraints to keep patients from falling. Bed railings are the most common restraints. They prevent patients from falling out of their beds. Nurses are vital parts of fall prevention programs and can help reduce the number of people falling and injuring themselves.

Words & Phrases

inpatient a patient who is staying at a hospital   **prevent** to keep; to stop something from happening   **alarm** a device that makes a loud sound to warn others   **restraint** a tool that stops a person from doing something   **vital** very important

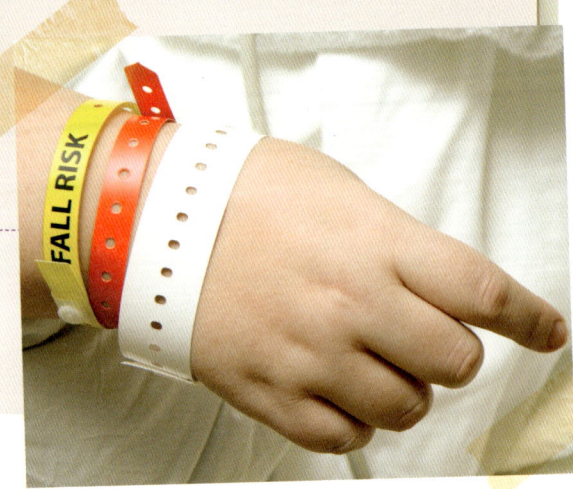

Basic Grammar

❶ prevent + 목적어 + from -ing   목적어가 ~하는 것을 방지하다

동사 prevent는 목적어 다음에 from -ing 형태를 취해, '목적어가 ~하는 것을 방지하다'라는 의미를 나타낸다.

You can set an alarm to prevent you from forgetting to take your pills.
약 드시는 것을 잊어버리는 것을 방지하도록 알람을 맞추어 놓으실 수 있습니다.

This will prevent you from scratching your scar.   이것이 상처를 긁는 것을 방지해 줄 겁니다.

❷ for instance   예를 들어

앞서 언급했던 것의 예를 들 때 사용하는 표현으로서, for example과 같은 의미를 나타낸다.

There are things you can do at home. For instance, you can do stretching exercises.
집에서 하실 수 있는 것들이 있습니다. 예를 들어, 스트레칭 운동을 하실 수 있습니다.

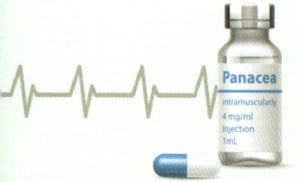

TIPS & TIPS

씻고 씻고 또 씻는 간호사의 손

간호사는 끊임없이 손을 씻습니다. 어떻게 보면 지나치다 싶을 정도지만, 간호사에게는 손을 청결하게 유지하는 것이 매우 중요하기 때문이지요. 간호사가 손을 씻는 방법은 이렇습니다. 먼저 비누를 사용해 손에 묻은 먼지나 이물질을 씻어냅니다. 그러고는 손 소독제를 이용하여 손에 남아 있는 다양한 세균과 병원균을 제거해 줍니다. 우리가 자주 사용하는 손과 손톱 밑에는 세균과 병원균이 득시글거리기 마련인데요. 간호사는 하루 종일 환자와 접촉하는 만큼, 자신의 손을 항상 청결하게 유지하는 데 신경 써야 합니다.

UNIT 09 Discussing Medication

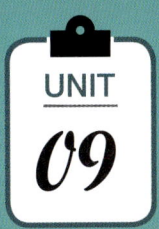

Warmup

다음은 어떤 약의 부작용에 대한 설명서입니다. 각 부작용을 사진에서 고르세요.

The Side Effects May Include:
1. sleep problems (insomnia) ☐
2. drowsiness, tired feeling ☐
3. stomach pain or upset ☐
4. dry eyes, blurred vision ☐

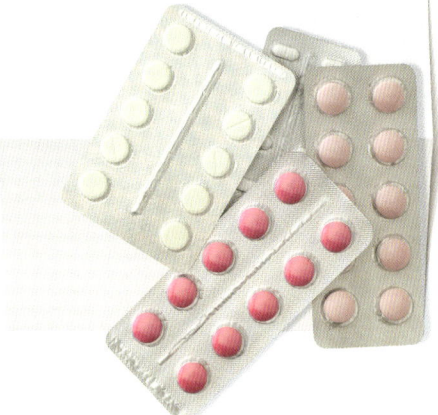
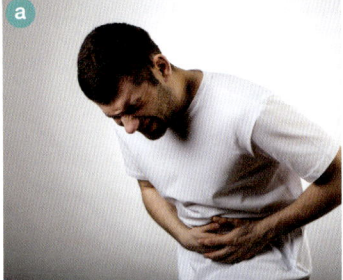
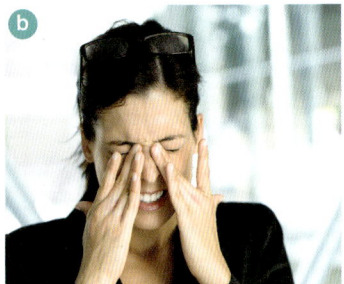
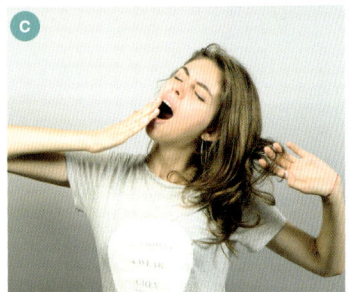
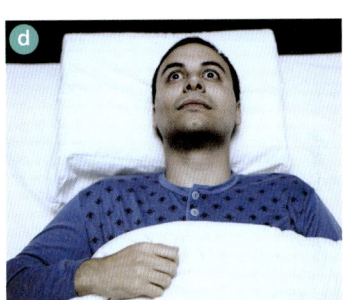

Vocabulary

주어진 의미에 어울리는 단어를 고르세요.

1. side effect •   • a. feeling like one has to throw up
2. drowsy •   • b. usually; regularly
3. nauseous •   • c. a lump; a mass
4. commonly •   • d. a minor problem caused by medicine
5. clot •   • e. sleepy

Track 49

Warmup Listening

문장을 듣고 그에 맞는 대답을 고르세요.

1. _____
   a. Will you give me a shot?   b. I feel better already.
2. _____
   a. You might feel sleepy.   b. The medicine is very effective.
3. _____
   a. There are seven of them.   b. These are pain relievers.

Unit 09 | 75

Conversation I

다음 대화를 듣고, 파트너와 함께 대화를 연습해 보세요.

Explaining the Possible Side Effects of Medication

Track 50

Nurse: Good afternoon, Mr. Walton. ¹It's time for your medication.
Patient: Good afternoon. Are you going to give me a shot?
Nurse: No, I'm not. ²I'm going to put your medication into the IV drip.
Patient: That's nice. I don't like needles.
Nurse: This medicine is going to make you feel a bit drowsy. In fact, you're probably going to fall asleep soon.
Patient: Are there any other side effects?
Nurse: ³You might feel a bit nauseous, and you may develop a skin rash. If either of these happens to you, please let me know. Then, the doctor can adjust your level of medication.
Patient: Okay, I'll do that. Wow, I already feel sleepy. I think I'm going to take a nap now.

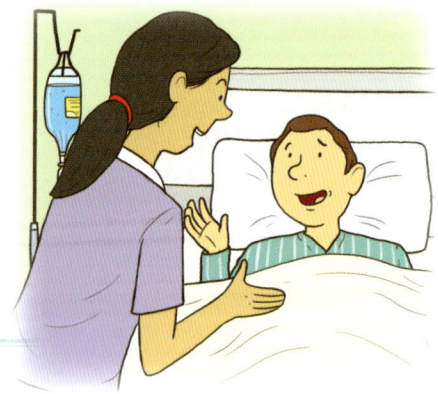

Key Expressions

❶ It's time for your medication. 약 (맞으실) 시간입니다.

환자에게 약을 맞거나 먹을 시간이라고 알릴 때 사용할 수 있는 표현으로, It's time for ~를 통해 무엇을 할 시간인지 나타낼 수 있다.

It's time for breakfast. 아침 드실 시간입니다.

❷ I'm going to put your medication into the IV drip. 약을 링거 주사로 투여해 드릴 겁니다.

환자에게 약을 링거 주사로 투여해 주겠다고 말하는 표현이다.

I will give you a shot. 주사를 놓을 겁니다.
Please take these pills orally. 이 알약들을 복용하세요.

❸ You might feel a bit nauseous, and you may develop a skin rash.
약간 메스꺼우실 수도 있으며, 피부 발진이 생기실 수도 있습니다.

환자에게 약물의 부작용 등에 대해 미리 설명해 줄 때 사용할 수 있다. 불확실한 추측이나 가능성을 나타내는 may나 might를 쓸 수 있다.

This might make you feel sleepy. 이 약을 드시면 졸음이 오실 수도 있습니다.
You may get a headache. 두통이 생기실 수도 있습니다.

Useful Phrases

약물의 부작용에 대해 설명하는 표현

You may feel a bit drowsy. 조금 졸리실 수도 있습니다.
You will feel a little dizzy [lightheaded]. 약간 어지러우실 겁니다.
This can cause constipation [diarrhea]. 변비[설사]가 생길 수 있습니다.
You might experience heartburn. 속 쓰림이 있을 수도 있습니다.
Some people experience skin reactions. 일부 환자는 피부 반응을 보이기도 합니다.

Basic Drills

A 주어진 문장에 어울리는 대답을 고르세요.

1. Are you going to give me a shot? •   • a. Okay, I'll do that.
2. Are there any other side effects? •   • b. You might feel a bit nauseous, and you may develop a skin rash.
3. If either of these happens to you, •   • c. I'm going to put your medication into the IV drip.
   please let me know.

B 괄호 안의 말을 순서대로 배열하여, 주어진 의미를 영어로 표현하세요.

1. 약 (맞으실) 시간입니다. (time / medication / it's / your / for)
   _____

2. 약을 링거 주사로 투여해 드릴 겁니다. (the IV drip / put / I'm going to / into / your medication)
   _____

3. 약간 메스꺼우실 수도 있으며, 피부 발진이 생기실 수도 있습니다.
   (a bit nauseous / you / and / a skin rash / you might feel / may develop)
   _____

Buildup Activities

대화를 듣고 빈칸을 채운 후, 주어진 질문에 답하세요.

 Track 51

Nurse	Good evening, Mr. Buford. I have to give you your (a)_____ now.
Patient	Good evening. You're not going to give me a (b)_____, are you?
Nurse	No, I'm not. I've got some (c)_____ for you to take.
Patient	Good. I don't like (d)_____ very much.
Nurse	This medicine is going to make you feel a bit sleepy. In fact, you're probably going to take a nap soon.
Patient	Does it have any other (e)_____?
Nurse	You might get a bit dizzy, and you (f)_____ a bit. Please tell me if either of these happens to you. Then, the doctor can adjust your level of medication.
Patient	Okay, I'll do that. Wow, I am already getting sleepy. I think I'm going to fall asleep now.

1. How does the nurse give the patient his medicine?
   a. by giving him a shot
   b. by putting it in his IV drip
   c. by giving him some pills

2. What is NOT a side effect of the medicine?
   a. nausea
   b. dizziness
   c. drowsiness

Conversation II

다음 대화를 듣고, 파트너와 함께 대화를 연습해 보세요.

Answering Patients' Questions about Medication

Track 52

Nurse	It's time to take your medicine, Mr. Peters.
Patient	That's a lot of pills. What do I need to take all of them for?
Nurse	¹These pills help prevent blood clots from forming. These ones will help lower your blood pressure. And this pill is pain medication. It'll help you experience less pain.
Patient	Is it safe to take so many pills at the same time?
Nurse	Yes, it is. ²Patients who have heart surgery commonly get all of these types of medicine.
Patient	Can I take them on an empty stomach?
Nurse	Absolutely not. You don't want to do that. They could upset your stomach, make you feel nauseous, or cause you to vomit.
Patient	What about the side effects of all these pills?
Nurse	³Let me bring you a sheet of paper. It describes the side effects of each medicine you're taking.

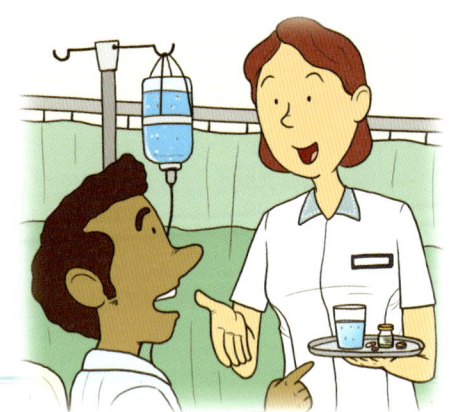

» Key Expressions

❶ These pills help prevent blood clots from forming.   이 알약들은 혈전이 생기는 것을 예방해 줍니다.

환자가 복용할 약이 어떤 기능을 하는지 안내하는 표현이다.

This is for muscle cramps.   이것은 근육 경련을 위한 것입니다.
These pills will reduce your fever.   이 알약들은 열을 내려 줄 겁니다.

❷ Patients who have heart surgery commonly get all of these types of medicine.

심장 수술을 받는 환자들은 보통 이런 종류의 약을 먹습니다.

여러 가지 약을 한꺼번에 먹어도 괜찮은지 걱정하는 환자를 안심시키는 표현이다.

❸ Let me bring you a sheet of paper.   제가 종이를 한 장 가져다 드리겠습니다.

약의 부작용에 대해 설명되어 있는 안내문을 가져다 주겠다고 하는 표현이다.

I will get you a copy of information about those pills.   그 알약들의 정보를 한 부 가져다 드리겠습니다.

Useful Phrases ✚

> 환자에게 어떤 행동을 삼가라는 표현

= You don't want to do that. 그러지 않는 게 좋을 겁니다.
= You shouldn't do that. 그러시면 안 됩니다.
= Try not to do that. 그렇게 하지 않도록 하세요.
= I wouldn't do that if I were you. 저라면 그렇게 하지 않겠습니다.
= It is better if you don't do that. 그러지 않는 편이 낫습니다.

Basic Drills

A 주어진 문장에 어울리는 대답을 고르세요.

1. What do I need to take all of them for?
2. Is it safe to take so many pills at the same time?
3. Can I take them on an empty stomach?

a. You don't want to do that.
b. These pills help prevent blood clots from forming.
c. Patients who have heart surgery commonly get all of these types of medicine.

B 괄호 안의 말을 순서대로 배열하여, 주어진 의미를 영어로 표현하세요.

1. 이 알약들은 혈전이 생기는 것을 예방해 줍니다. (forming / prevent / help / these pills / blood clots / from)

2. 심장 수술을 받는 환자들은 보통 이런 종류의 약을 먹습니다.
   (have heart surgery / medicine / patients who / all of these types of / commonly get)

3. 제가 종이를 한 장 가져다 드리겠습니다. (you / me / let / paper / bring / a sheet of)

Buildup Activities

대화를 듣고 빈칸을 채운 후, 주어진 질문에 답하세요.

Track 53

Nurse	It's time for your medicine, Mr. Marino.
Patient	That's a lot (a)_____. What are they all for?
Nurse	These pills will keep (b)_____ from developing. This medication will help decrease your blood pressure. And this one is a pain reliever. It will stop your body from hurting so much.
Patient	Is it (c)_____ so many pills at once?
Nurse	Yes, it is. Organ transplant patients usually get all of these kinds of medicine.
Patient	Is it okay to take them on an (d)_____?
Nurse	Absolutely not. You shouldn't do that. They could give you a stomachache, make you feel (e)_____, or make you throw up.
Patient	What about the side effects of all this medicine?
Nurse	I will bring you a pamphlet in a minute. It (f)_____ the side effects of each medicine you're taking.

1. What kind of operation did the patient have?
   a. heart surgery
   b. an organ transplant
   c. brain surgery

2. What will the nurse bring the patient?
   a. a sheet of paper
   b. a book
   c. a pamphlet

Job Simulation I

A 〈보기〉에서 적절한 말을 찾아, 각 그림의 상황에 맞는 대화를 완성하세요.

> 보기
> I'm going to put your medication in your IV drip.
> It's time for you to take your medicine.
> You may feel nauseous or develop a rash on your skin.

1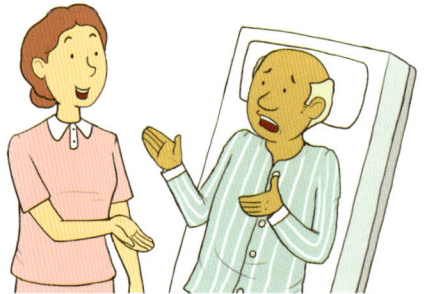
_____

How are you going to give it to me?

2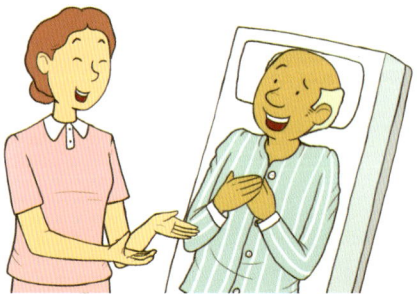
_____

Great. I don't like getting shots.

3 Does the medicine have any other side effects?

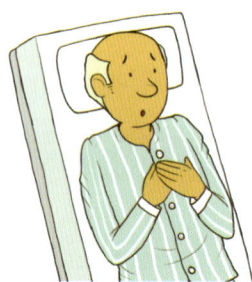 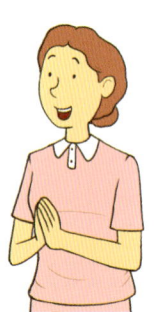

_____

B 주어진 세 가지 상황을 이용하여, 파트너와 함께 각 상황에 맞는 대화를 연습해 보세요.

Situation	(a)	(b)
1	very sleepy	get some acne
2	really tired	have some bad headaches
3	rather drowsy	experience some muscle or joint pain

Nurse   This medicine is going to make you feel (a)_____. In fact, you're probably going to fall asleep soon.

Patient   Are there any other side effects?

Nurse   You might feel a bit nauseous, and you may (b)_____. If either of these happens to you, please let me know.

80 | Discussing Medication

Job Simulation II

A 〈보기〉에서 적절한 말을 찾아, 각 그림의 상황에 맞는 대화를 완성하세요.

> 보기
> I'll bring you a sheet of paper that explains all of them.
> Liver transplant patients usually have to take these.
> These pills will help prevent your body from getting infected.

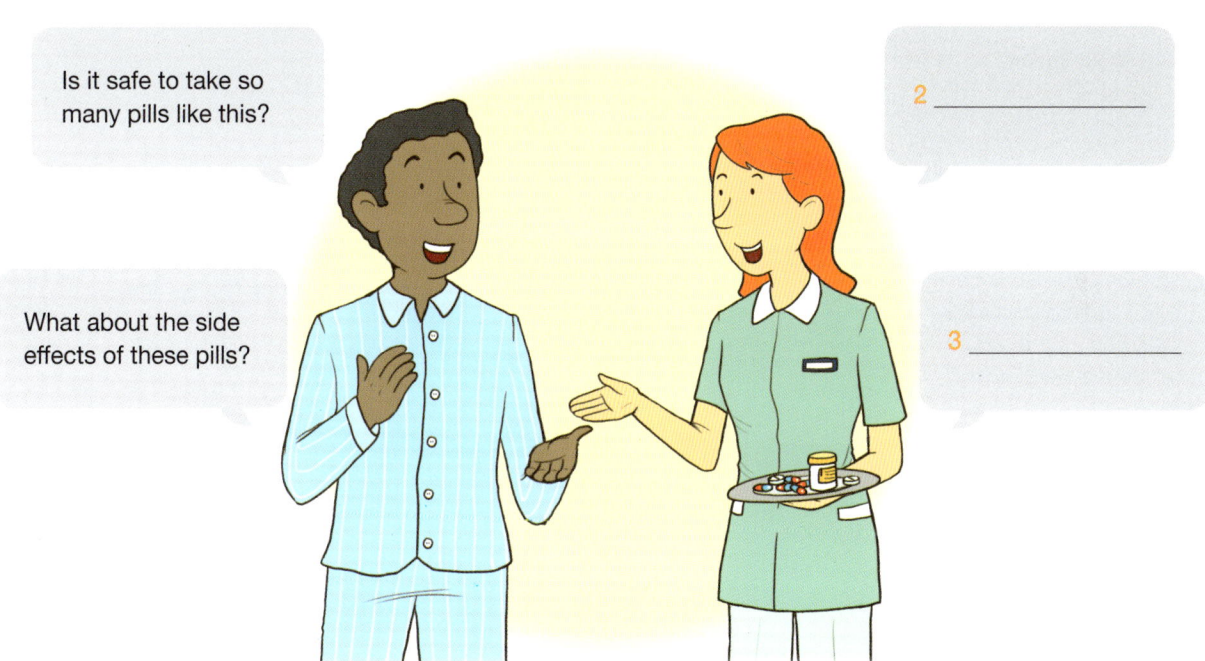

Why do I have to take these pills?

1 _____

Is it safe to take so many pills like this?

2 _____

What about the side effects of these pills?

3 _____

B 주어진 세 가지 상황을 이용하여, 파트너와 함께 각 상황에 맞는 대화를 연습해 보세요.

Situation	(a)	(b)	(c)
1	stop blood clots from developing	all of these pills together	need all of this medicine
2	keep your heart strong	so much medication at one time	have to take this much medicine
3	keep your body safe from infection	this large amount of pills right now	won't get better without all these pills

Patient That's a lot of pills. What do I need to take all of them for?

Nurse These pills help (a)_____. These ones will help lower your blood pressure. And this pill is pain medication. It'll help you experience less pain.

Patient Is it safe to take (b)_____?

Nurse Yes, it is. Patients who have heart surgery (c)_____.

Reading & Listening

다음 지문을 읽고, 음성을 들어 보세요.

Preventing Medication Errors

Track 54

Every year, millions of people around the world receive the wrong medicine. Many of these people develop severe problems, and some even die. Nurses must be careful not ¹to make any medication errors with their patients. First, they ²should carefully read all the information about their patients and their medications. Good communication is important as well. Nurses must communicate with other nurses and doctors about what medicine their patients are getting, how much they are getting, and when they are getting it. Nurses should closely read the labels on medication. Some medicines look the same or have similar packaging, so it is easy to mix them up. Nurses should also diligently monitor their patients to see how they react to the medicine. They should explain what each medication does to their patients and listen carefully when patients report problems. By following these steps, nurses can help prevent medication errors.

Words & Phrases

error a mistake   **packaging** the package or container that a product comes in   **mix up** to confuse; to make a mistake   **diligently** carefully   **react** to respond to something

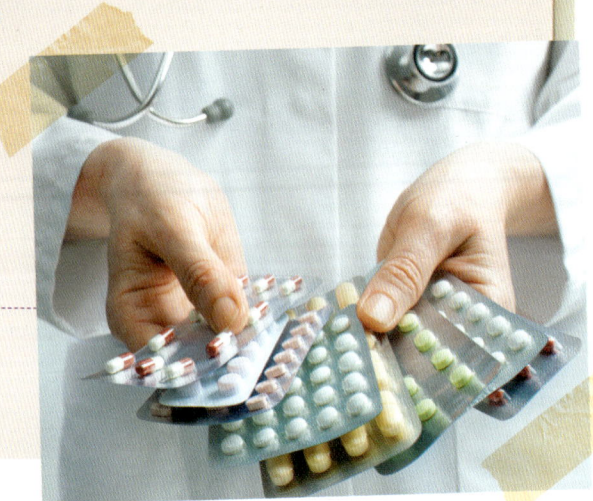

Basic Grammar

❶ to부정사의 부사적 용법

to부정사는 문장에서 동사, 형용사, 부사 등의 역할을 한다. 본문에서는 to부정사가 부사의 역할을 하여 목적의 의미를 나타냈다.

Mrs. Watson pushed the button to call a nurse.   Watson 부인은 간호사를 부르기 위해 버튼을 눌렀다.

❷ '의무'를 나타내는 조동사 should

조동사 should는 '~해야 한다'라는 뜻으로 도덕적 의무나, 어떤 것을 당연히 해야 함을 나타낼 때 사용한다. ought to도 같은 의미이다.

You should talk to the doctor about your rash.   발진에 관해서는 의사 선생님께 말씀하셔야 합니다.
You ought to call us in advance if you are not able to keep your appointment.
진료 예약을 지키실 수 없다면 미리 저희에게 전화해 주셔야 합니다.

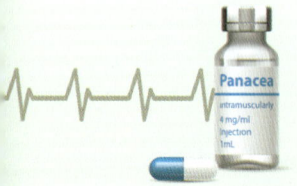

TIPS&TIPS

환자가 'ER'에서 올라왔다고요?

"CBC 검사 결과 떴습니다." "IV로 드리는 건가요?" "이전 처방 D/C해 주세요." "ER에서 환자분 올라오셨습니다."
병원 의료진 사이에서는 이 같은 대화가 흔히 오갑니다. 대화 중에 약어가 자주 등장하는 만큼, 간호사는 각 약어가 무슨 뜻인지 정확히 알고 있어야 합니다. CBC는 Complete Blood Count의 약어로 '전혈구검사'를 뜻하며, IV는 Intravenous 의 약어로 '정맥주사'를 뜻합니다. 또한 D/C는 Discontinue의 약어로 '중단'을 의미하며, ER은 Emergency Room의 약어로 '응급실'을 의미하지요.

Discussing Medication

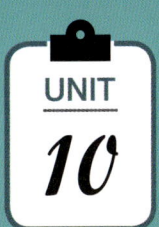

UNIT 10
Reassuring Patients and Guardians

Warmup
다음 사진을 마취 수술이 진행되는 순서대로 배열해 보세요.

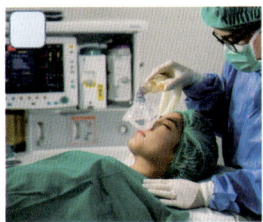
The patient inhales anesthetic gas.

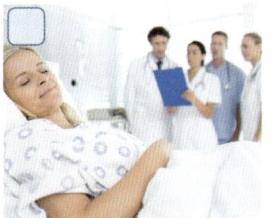
The patient is sent to the recovery room.

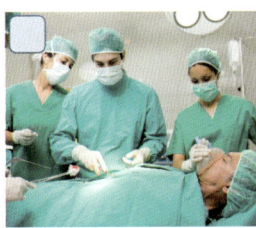
The patient has surgery.

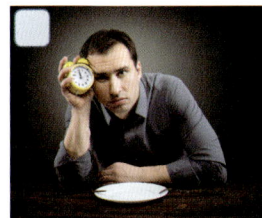
The patient fasts for hours.

Vocabulary
주어진 의미에 어울리는 단어를 고르세요.

1. groggy
2. wear off
3. complication
4. anesthesia
5. surgeon

a. a doctor who performs surgeries
b. sleepy; weak; unsteady
c. the use of medicine that prevents a person from experiencing pain
d. to stop having an effect on the body
e. a difficulty; a problem

Warmup Listening
문장을 듣고 그에 맞는 대답을 고르세요.

Track 55

1.
   a. I'm a bit sore.
   b. Please feel my forehead.
2.
   a. It's a complicated answer.
   b. The surgery was successful.
3.
   a. She's in the recovery room.
   b. Yes, you have seen her.

Conversation I

다음 대화를 듣고, 파트너와 함께 대화를 연습해 보세요.

Reassuring Patients Waking Up from Surgery

Track 56

Patient	Oh . . . Where . . . Where am I?
Nurse	Ah, you're finally awake. ¹Can you tell me your name?
Patient	My name . . . ? Yeah, I'm Eric Martin.
Nurse	Very good, Mr. Martin.
Patient	Where am I?
Nurse	You're in the hospital's recovery room right now. Your surgery is over. ²How do you feel? Can you open your eyes?
Patient	I feel a little groggy. I'm trying to open my eyes, but . . .
Nurse	³You feel that way because of the anesthesia. It will wear off soon. Are you in pain?
Patient	Yeah, my chest hurts a bit. My throat is really dry. Can I have some water?
Nurse	Not yet. You've got to wait a while before you can drink anything.

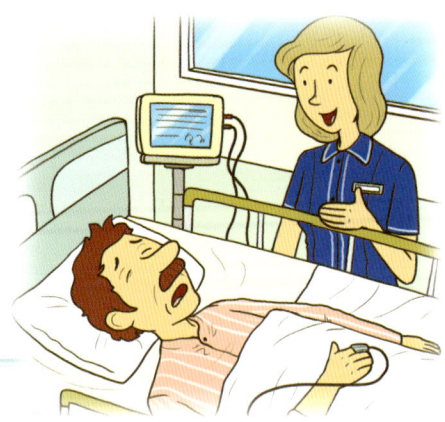

» Key Expressions

❶ Can you tell me your name?   환자분 성함을 말씀해 보시겠어요?

전신 마취나 수면 마취 수술 후 환자의 의식이 어느 정도 돌아왔는지 확인하기 위해 본인의 이름을 말해 보라고 하는 표현이다.

Can you tell me where you are?   여기가 어딘지 말씀해 보시겠어요?
Can you tell me who I am?   제가 누군지 말씀해 보시겠어요?
Can you rate your pain on a scale of 0 to 10?   통증의 정도가 0점에서 10점까지 중 몇 점이세요?

❷ How do you feel?   좀 어떠세요?

환자의 컨디션을 물을 때 사용할 수 있는 표현이다.

How are you feeling?   좀 어떠세요?

❸ You feel that way because of the anesthesia.   마취 때문에 그렇게 느끼시는 겁니다.

수술을 끝낸 환자의 정신이 혼미하거나(groggy), 어지럽거나(dizzy), 혼란스러운(confused) 것은 마취 때문이라고 말하는 표현이다.

The reason is that the anesthesia hasn't worn off yet.   마취가 아직 안 풀려서 그렇습니다.
It is connected with the medicine you had earlier.   좀 전에 드신 약과 관련이 있습니다.

Useful Phrases ➕

> 환자가 통증을 느끼는지 확인하는 표현

Are you in pain?   아프세요?
Are you experiencing any pain?   어디 아프세요?
Are you having any pain or discomfort right now?   지금 어디 아프시거나 불편하신 데 있으세요?

Basic Drills

A 주어진 문장에 어울리는 대답을 고르세요.

1. Can you tell me your name?   •   • a. You're in the hospital's recovery room right now.
2. Where am I?   •   • b. Yeah, I'm Eric Martin.
3. I feel a little groggy.   •   • c. You feel that way because of the anesthesia.

B 괄호 안의 말을 순서대로 배열하여, 주어진 의미를 영어로 표현하세요.

1. 환자분 성함을 말씀해 보시겠어요? (tell / you / can / me / your name)
   _____

2. 좀 어떠세요? (feel / you / how / do)
   _____

3. 마취 때문에 그렇게 느끼시는 겁니다. (the anesthesia / you / that way / feel / because of)
   _____

Buildup Activities

대화를 듣고 빈칸을 채운 후, 주어진 질문에 답하세요.

Patient	Oh . . . Where . . . Where am I?
Nurse	Ah, you're (a)_____. Do you know your name?
Patient	My name . . . ? Yeah, I'm Peter Robinson.
Nurse	Well done, Mr. Robinson.
Patient	Can you tell me (b)_____ I am?
Nurse	You're in the (c)_____ at Central Hospital. Your operation went well. How are you feeling? Why don't you try to open your eyes?
Patient	I (d)_____. I want to open my eyes, but I can't.
Nurse	That will be hard to do for a while because of the anesthesia. Do you have any pain?
Patient	(e)_____ hurts really badly. And my throat is dry. Can I get a drink of water?
Nurse	Not yet. You're not allowed to drink anything for (f)_____.

1. How does the patient feel?
   a. great
   b. awful
   c. sleepy

2. When can the patient get some water?
   a. now
   b. in 20 minutes
   c. in an hour

Conversation II

다음 대화를 듣고, 파트너와 함께 대화를 연습해 보세요.

Reassuring Patients' Guardians

Guardian: How did Lucy's surgery go? Were there any complications?
Nurse: ¹Everything worked out fine, sir. Your daughter's surgeon will come here to tell you about it in five minutes.
Guardian: Can I see her now?
Nurse: ²She's still in the recovery room and hasn't woken up yet. You'll have to wait a while.
Guardian: When is she going to wake up?
Nurse: She should be awake in around twenty minutes. You can visit her in her room an hour from now.
Guardian: All right. That sounds fine.
Nurse: ³Why don't you sit down and relax? Dr. Kim will be with you in a moment.

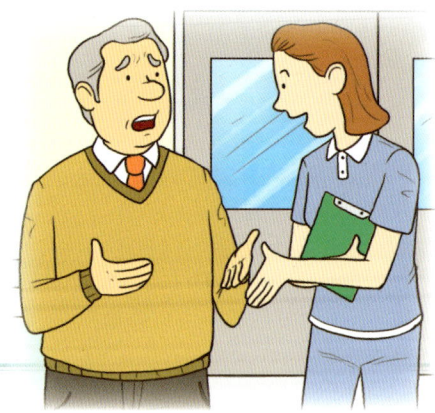

Key Expressions

❶ Everything worked out fine. 다 잘되었습니다.

환자의 보호자에게 수술이 잘되었다고 말하는 표현이다. work out fine 대신에 go well(잘되다)이나, be successful(성공적이다)을 사용할 수도 있다.

Everything went very well. 다 매우 잘됐습니다.
The surgery was successful. 수술은 성공적이었습니다.

❷ She's still in the recovery room and hasn't woken up yet. 따님은 아직 회복실에 있는데, 아직 깨어나지 않았습니다.

환자가 수술 후 아직 깨어나지 않았다는 표현을 할 때 사용한다. not wake up(깨어나지 않다) 대신에 be under anesthesia(마취 상태에 있다)나 not come out of anesthesia(마취에서 깨어나지 않다)도 같은 의미를 나타낼 때 사용할 수 있다.

She is still under anesthesia. 그녀는 아직 마취 상태에 있습니다.
The patient hasn't come out of anesthesia yet. 환자는 아직 마취에서 깨어나지 않았습니다.

❸ Why don't you sit down and relax? 앉아서 쉬시는 게 어때요?

환자가 깨어나기를 기다리는 보호자에게 잠시 앉아서 쉬기를 제안하는 표현이다. How [What] about ~?도 제안이나 권유를 할 때 사용할 수 있다.

How about taking a seat here? 여기 앉는 게 어떠세요?
Please have a seat and try to relax. 여기 앉아서 좀 쉬세요.

Useful Phrases

| You'll have to V ~하셔야 할 것입니다. |

You'll have to wait a while. 좀 기다리셔야 할 것입니다.
You'll have to sign a consent form before surgery. 수술 전에 동의서에 서명하셔야 할 것입니다.
You'll have to take off all your clothes and put on this gown. 옷을 전부 벗으시고 이 가운을 입으셔야 할 것입니다.
You'll have to avoid high-fiber foods and raw vegetables. 섬유질이 풍부한 식품과 생채소를 피하셔야 할 것입니다.

Basic Drills

A 주어진 문장에 어울리는 대답을 고르세요.

1. When is she going to wake up? •   • a. She should be awake in around twenty minutes.
2. How did Lucy's surgery go?   •   • b. Everything worked out fine.
3. Can I see her now?   •   • c. You'll have to wait a while.

B 괄호 안의 말을 순서대로 배열하여, 주어진 의미를 영어로 표현하세요.

1. 다 잘되었습니다. (worked / fine / out / everything)
   _____

2. 따님은 아직 회복실에 있는데, 아직 깨어나지 않았습니다.
   (still / and / woken up yet / hasn't / she's / in the recovery room)
   _____

3. 앉아서 쉬시는 게 어때요? (don't / and / you / relax / why / sit down)
   _____

Buildup Activities

대화를 듣고 빈칸을 채운 후, 주어진 질문에 답하세요.

 Track 59

Guardian	How was Gina Gilman's (a)_____? Were there any problems?
Nurse	The operation was successful, sir. (b)_____ surgeon will speak with you about it in a moment.
Guardian	Can I (c)_____ her now?
Nurse	She's still sleeping in the recovery room. You have to wait until she wakes up.
Guardian	When will she be (d)_____?
Nurse	She will probably wake up in about (e)_____. You can see her in her room in an hour or so.
Guardian	Okay. Thank you.
Nurse	How about (f)_____ and relaxing a bit? Dr. Wilson will be here soon.

1. Who had surgery?

   a. the man's wife

   b. the man's sister

   c. the man's daughter

2. When will the patient wake up?

   a. in 10 minutes

   b. in 30 minutes

   c. in 1 hour

Job Simulation I

A 〈보기〉에서 적절한 말을 찾아, 각 그림의 상황에 맞는 대화를 완성하세요.

> 보기
> How do you feel?
> Can you remember your name?
> The anesthesia is making you feel that way.

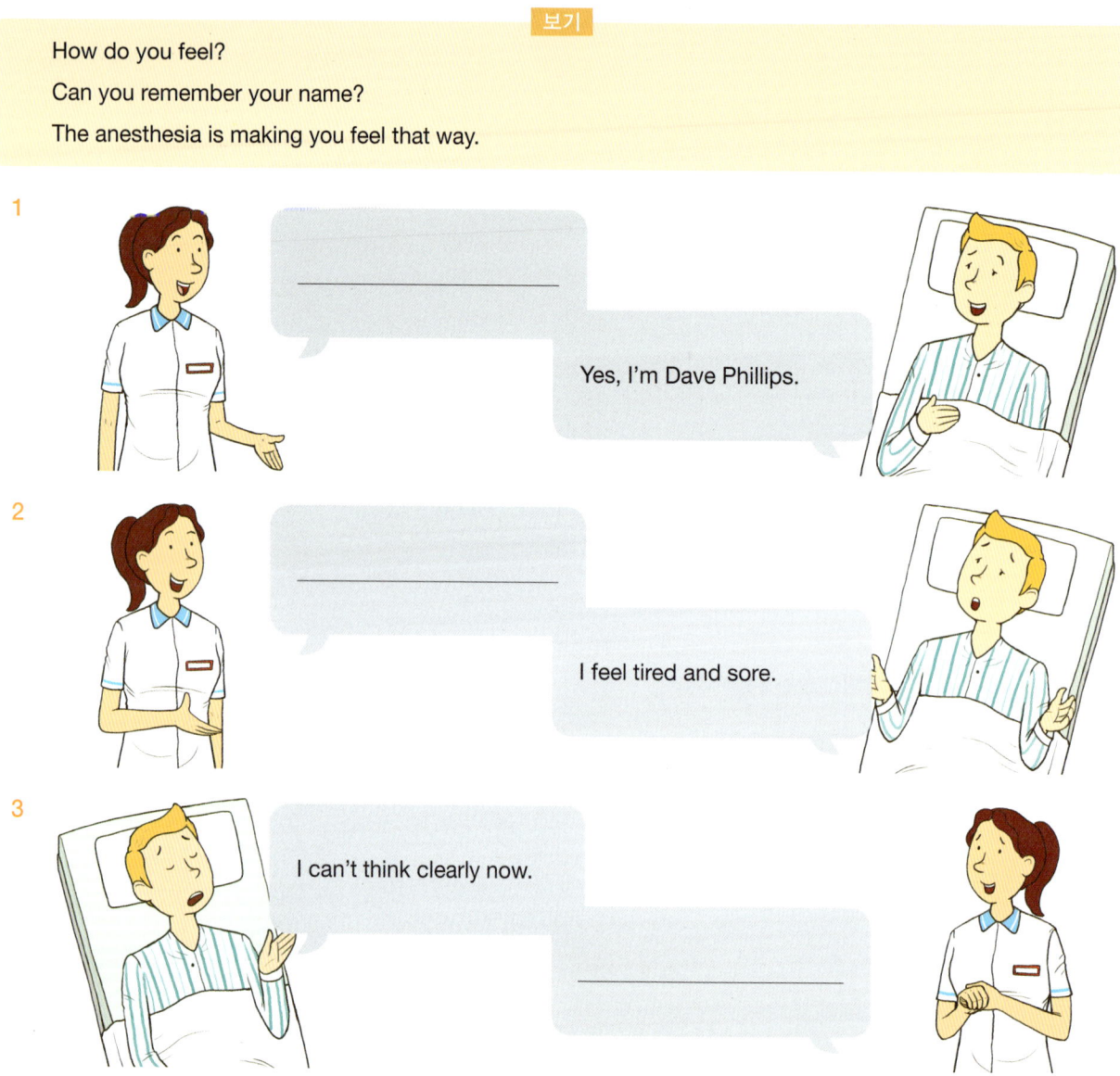

1. _____
   Yes, I'm Dave Phillips.

2. _____
   I feel tired and sore.

3. I can't think clearly now.
   _____

B 주어진 세 가지 상황을 이용하여, 파트너와 함께 각 상황에 맞는 대화를 연습해 보세요.

Situation	(a)	(b)	(c)
1	lightheaded	in pain	get a drink of water
2	like someone hit me on the head with a hammer	feeling any pain	have a glass of water
3	terrible	sore anywhere	get something to drink

Nurse	How do you feel? Can you open your eyes?
Patient	I feel (a)_____. I'm trying to open my eyes, but . . .
Nurse	You feel that way because of the anesthesia. Are you (b)_____?
Patient	Yeah, my chest hurts a bit. My throat is really dry. Can I (c)_____?
Nurse	Not yet. You've got to wait a while before you can drink anything.

Reassuring Patients and Guardians

Job Simulation II

A 〈보기〉에서 적절한 말을 찾아, 각 그림의 상황에 맞는 대화를 완성하세요.

> 보기
>
> How about sitting down and relaxing for a bit?
> The operation was 100% successful.
> She's still sleeping in the recovery room.

1

How was the surgery?

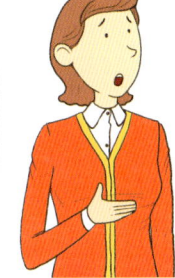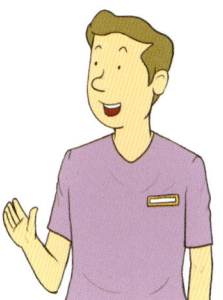

_____

2

Can I see my daughter now?

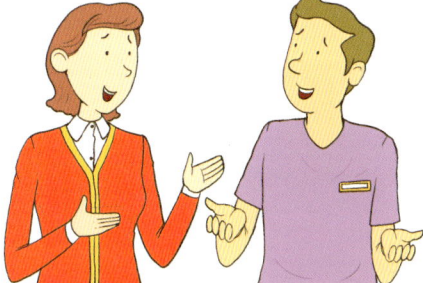

_____

3

I really want to see her soon.

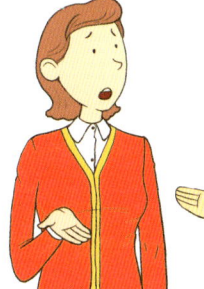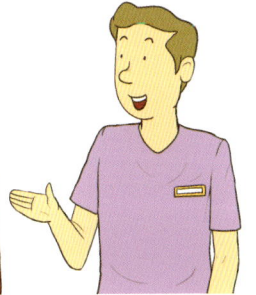

_____

B 주어진 세 가지 상황을 이용하여, 파트너와 함께 각 상황에 맞는 대화를 연습해 보세요.

Situation	(a)	(b)	(c)
1	Was everything all right	speak with you in a moment	isn't awake yet
2	Were there any problems during it	tell you about it momentarily	can't see anyone right now
3	Did everything go well	discuss it with you in a few minutes	needs to wake up first

Visitor   How did Lucy's surgery go? (a)_____?

Nurse   Everything worked out fine, sir. Your daughter's surgeon will come here to (b)_____.

Visitor   Can I see her now?

Nurse   She's still in the recovery room and (c)_____. You'll have to wait a while.

Reading & Listening

다음 지문을 읽고, 음성을 들어 보세요.

Therapeutic Relationships between Nurses and Patients

Track 60

Nurses spend a great deal of time with patients. For that reason, they must develop good relationships with their patients. That will [1]enable their patients to get the best care possible and to recover quickly. There are three important aspects to a therapeutic relationship: physical, psychological, and emotional care. Nurses must work closely with their patients to set goals for their physical improvement. Then, they must make sure their patients meet those goals and constantly improve. Nurses need to have good communication with their patients to provide good psychological and emotional care. This does not just involve speaking. It requires listening and body language, too. Nurses must [2]show their patients that they care and are interested in their patients' well-being. They should have empathy for their patients as well. Finally, by earning the trust and respect of their patients, nurses can provide the best care possible.

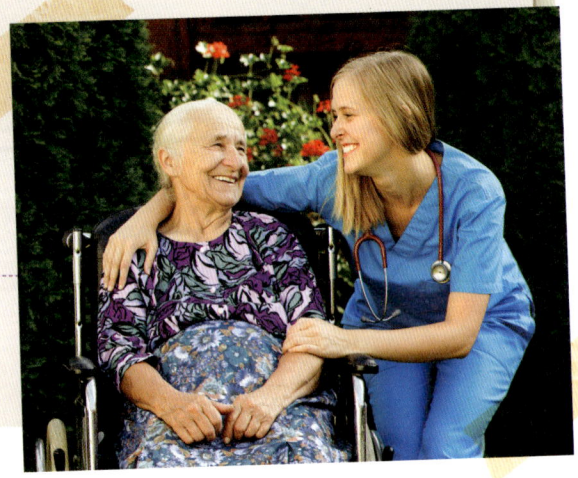

Words & Phrases

therapeutic healing **psychological** relating to the mind **meet a goal** to be successful in one's objective **empathy** the ability to feel sympathy for others **earn one's trust** to make another person believe or trust in oneself

» Basic Grammar

① enable + 목적어 + to V 목적어가 ~할 수 있게 해 주다

동사 enable이 목적격 보어로 to부정사를 취하면 '목적어가 ~할 수 있게 해 주다'라는 의미를 나타낸다.

This will enable you to walk more comfortably. 이것이 더 편하게 걸을 수 있게 해 줄 겁니다.
Anesthesia enables a patient to tolerate surgical procedures. 마취는 환자가 수술 과정을 견딜 수 있게 해 준다.

② 4형식 동사 show

동사 show는 'show + 간접목적어+ 직접목적어'의 형식을 취하는 4형식 동사로 쓰일 수 있다. 이때 의미는 '(간접목적어)에게 (직접목적어)를 보여 주다'가 된다. 본문의 show처럼 직접목적어 자리에 that절이 올 수 있는 4형식 동사에는 tell, inform, remind 등이 있다.

The nurse told him that he needed to sit up straight. 간호사는 그에게 똑바로 앉아야 한다고 말했다.
The doctor informed the patient that she could go home. 의사는 환자에게 퇴원해도 된다고 알렸다.
The nurse reminded her that there might be side effects. 간호사는 부작용이 있을 수도 있다는 것을 그녀에게 상기시켜 주었다.

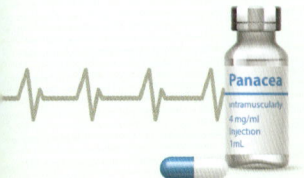

TIPS & TIPS

'전인 간호'란 무엇인가요?

정확히 무슨 뜻인지 모르고도 사람들이 무심코 쓰는 말 중 하나가 '전인 간호'가 아닐까 싶습니다. 전인 간호란 환자의 신체만을 돌보는 것이 아니라, 더 나아가 환자의 몸과 마음, 그리고 영혼까지 돌보는 간호를 말합니다. 예를 들면, 필요한 말만 하고 뒤돌아서기보다는 시간이 조금 더 걸리더라도 환자의 말에 끝까지 귀를 기울이고, 환자를 진심으로 대하는 거지요. 또한 환자가 자라온 문화적 배경이나 종교 등을 비롯한 환자 개개인의 특성에 맞추어 환자를 간호하고자 노력하는 것입니다.

UNIT 11 Discharging Patients

Warmup
다음은 허리 디스크 환자의 퇴원 후 주의사항입니다. 주의사항을 어긴 환자를 사진에서 모두 찾아 보세요.

Guidelines after Leaving the Hospital

- Avoid smoking and drinking.
- Don't exercise too much.
- Be careful bending over.
- Eat healthy food.

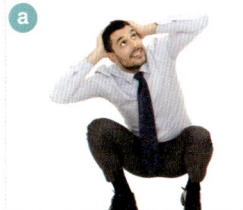
a

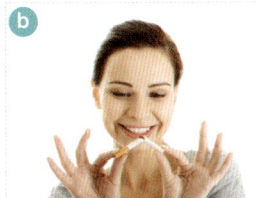
b

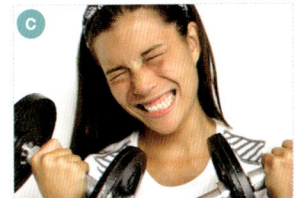
c

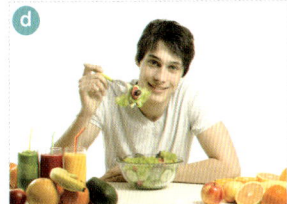
d

Vocabulary
주어진 의미에 어울리는 단어를 고르세요.

1. records
2. definitely
3. be responsible for
4. bill
5. stride

- a. to have to do something
- b. for sure; absolutely
- c. information preserved in writing
- d. a step
- e. a statement of money owed for a service

Track 61

Warmup Listening
문장을 듣고 그에 맞는 대답을 고르세요.

1.
   a. Okay, I will.   b. This is my prescription.
2.
   a. Yes, here is your card.   b. No, we have that information.
3.
   a. Yes, I paid my bill.   b. I'll use cash.

Conversation I

다음 대화를 듣고, 파트너와 함께 대화를 연습해 보세요.

Informing Patients of Dos and Don'ts Track 62

Nurse	You're being discharged from the hospital, Mr. Grimes, but you have a few things to do at home.
Patient	Yes? What are they?
Nurse	¹Be sure to take your medication three times a day. Do that thirty minutes after you eat. Please don't forget to take it.
Patient	All right. I'll definitely take it every day.
Nurse	²If you have to cough, press a pillow against your abdomen. That will help ease the pain.
Patient	What about walking?
Nurse	Be careful when you walk. ³Don't take long strides. Instead, take short steps.
Patient	Thank you for the information.

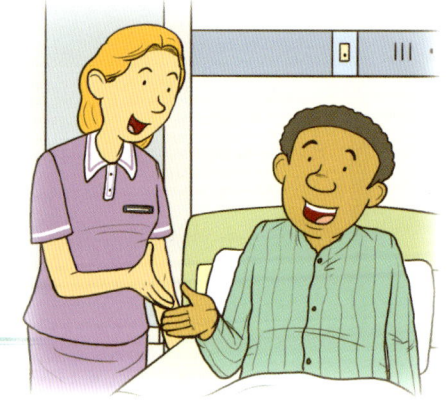

» Key Expressions

❶ Be sure to take your medication three times a day. 약은 하루에 세 번 꼭 드세요.

be [make] sure ~(꼭 ~ 하다)를 사용하여 환자에게 약을 잘 챙겨먹으라고 당부할 수 있다.

You should take these pills every 4 hours. 이 알약들을 4시간마다 드셔야 합니다.
Don't forget to take those after each meal. 식후마다 그것들을 드시는 것을 잊지 마세요.

❷ If you have to cough, press a pillow against your abdomen. 기침이 나오면, 베개로 배를 누르세요.

기침을 해야 한다면 베개로 배를 누르라고 설명하는 표현이다.

When you cough, try to push a pillow against your tummy. 기침을 하실 때는, 베개로 배를 누르세요.
If you have to lift something, use your knees. Don't bend over. 어떤 것을 들어야 하면, 무릎을 사용하세요. 허리를 숙이지 마시고요.

❸ Don't take long strides. 큰 보폭으로 걷지 마세요.

환자가 해서는 안 되는 행동을 Don't ~(~하지 마세요)를 사용해 설명하는 표현이다. should not이나, try not to V를 사용하여 환자가 피해야 할 행동을 설명할 수도 있다.

You should not run. 뛰시면 안 됩니다.
Try not to walk fast. Walk slowly. 빨리 걷지 마세요. 천천히 걸으세요.

Useful Phrases

환자에게 퇴원을 알리는 표현

You're being discharged from the hospital. 병원에서 퇴원하실 겁니다.
You're going to be discharged next week. 다음 주에 퇴원하실 겁니다.
You can go home either today or tomorrow. 오늘이나 내일 퇴원하실 수 있습니다.
You may leave the hospital. 퇴원하셔도 됩니다.

Basic Drills

A 주어진 문장에 어울리는 대답을 고르세요.

1. You have a few things to do at home.   •   • a. Don't take long strides.
2. What about walking?   •   • b. I'll definitely take it every day.
3. Be sure to take your medication three times a day.   •   • c. Yes? What are they?

B 괄호 안의 말을 순서대로 배열하여, 주어진 의미를 영어로 표현하세요.

1. 약은 하루에 세 번 꼭 드세요. (be sure to / a day / your medication / three times / take)

   _____

2. 기침이 나오면, 베개로 배를 누르세요. (have to cough / against / a pillow / if you / your abdomen / press)

   _____

3. 큰 보폭으로 걷지 마세요. (don't / strides / long / take)

   _____

Buildup Activities

대화를 듣고 빈칸을 채운 후, 주어진 질문에 답하세요.

Nurse   You're being (a)_____ today, Mr. Wake, but you still have several things to do at home.

Patient   Okay, what kinds of things?

Nurse   You have to take your medicine daily. Take it (b)_____ a day after meals. Be sure you take all your pills.

Patient   Don't worry. I'll take all of (c)_____.

Nurse   Whenever you cough, hold (d)_____ against your stomach. That will make you feel less pain.

Patient   What about when I (e)_____?

Nurse   Be very careful. Don't walk fast. Instead, you should (f)_____.

Patient   I'll be sure to remember that.

1. How often does the patient have to take his medicine?
   a. one time a day
   b. two times a day
   c. three times a day

2. What does the nurse tell the patient about walking?
   a. He can walk fast.
   b. He should not walk.
   c. He needs to walk slowly.

Conversation II

다음 대화를 듣고, 파트너와 함께 대화를 연습해 보세요.

Helping Patients Pay Their Bills

Track 64

Receptionist	Here's your bill, Ms. Weathers.
Patient	Thank you. Do you want to see my insurance card?
Receptionist	No, I don't. ¹We already have that information in our records.
Patient	How much is my insurance paying for this visit?
Receptionist	²Your insurance is covering fifty percent of the cost. You are responsible for the rest. ³How would you like to pay for that?
Patient	I don't have enough cash on me, so can I use a credit card?
Receptionist	Yes, you can.
Patient	Here you are.
Receptionist	Thank you. Sign here, please . . . And here is your receipt.

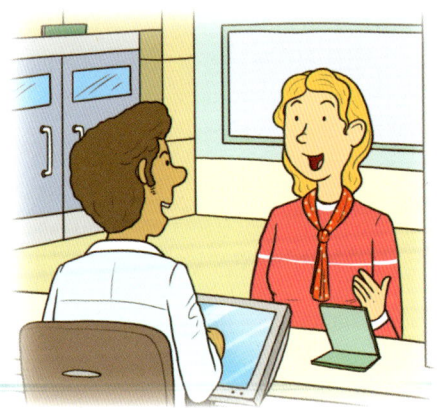

Key Expressions

❶ **We already have that information in our records.**   그 정보는 이미 저희 기록에 있습니다.

이미 병원에서 환자에 대한 특정 정보를 보유하고 있다는 의미로 사용한다.

You don't have to show your insurance card.   보험 카드는 보여 주지 않으셔도 됩니다.

❷ **Your insurance is covering fifty percent of the cost.**   환자분의 보험은 비용의 50퍼센트를 보장해 줄 것입니다.

병원비 중 얼마가 보험으로 처리되는지 안내하는 표현이다. 동사 cover는 '보장하다'라는 뜻으로 사용되었다.

Half of the cost is covered.   비용의 반이 보장됩니다.
You need to pay $35, and your insurance will take care of the rest.   35달러는 환자분께서 지불하셔야 하고, 나머지가 보험에서 처리됩니다.

❸ **How would you like to pay for that?**   그것을 어떻게 결제하시겠어요?

환자에게 병원비를 어떻게 결제할지 묻는 표현이다.

Would you like to pay for it by credit card?   그것을 신용카드로 계산하시겠어요?
We accept all major credit cards, checks, and cash.   저희는 모든 주요 신용카드, 수표 그리고 현금을 받습니다.

Useful Phrases

어떤 것을 건네줄 때 쓰는 표현

Here's your bill.   여기 계산서입니다.
This is your prescription.   여기 처방전입니다.
I will prepare your bill and prescription.   계산서와 처방전을 준비해 드리겠습니다.
Let me get you an appointment card.   예약 카드를 드리겠습니다.

Discharging Patients

Basic Drills

A 주어진 문장에 어울리는 대답을 고르세요.

1. How would you like to pay for that? •   • a. Can I use a credit card?
2. Do you want to see my insurance card? •   • b. Your insurance is covering fifty percent of the cost.
3. How much is my insurance paying for this visit? • • c. No, I don't.

B 괄호 안의 말을 순서대로 배열하여, 주어진 의미를 영어로 표현하세요.

1. 그 정보는 이미 저희 기록에 있습니다. (that information / we / in / our records / already have)

   _____

2. 환자분의 보험은 비용의 50퍼센트를 보장해 줄 것입니다. (the cost / your insurance / of / is covering / fifty percent)

   _____

3. 그것을 어떻게 결제하시겠어요? (you / like to pay / how / would / for that)

   _____

Buildup Activities

대화를 듣고 빈칸을 채운 후, 주어진 질문에 답하세요.   Track 65

Receptionist	This is (a)_____, Ms. Patterson.
Patient	Thank you. Would you like (b)_____ my insurance card?
Receptionist	That's all right. We have your insurance (c)_____ on file already.
Patient	How much does my insurance pay this time?
Receptionist	It's covering (d)_____ of the cost. You have to pay the rest. How are you going to pay today?
Patient	I didn't go to (e)_____ today, so I need to pay with a credit card.
Receptionist	That's fine.
Patient	Here it is.
Receptionist	Thank you . . . Sign here, please . . . And this is (f)_____.

1. How much is the patient's insurance covering?
   a. 40%   b. 50%   c. 60%

2. Why will the patient pay with her credit card?
   a. She did not go to the ATM.
   b. She has not gotten paid yet.
   c. She forgot to bring enough cash.

Job Simulation I

A 〈보기〉에서 적절한 말을 찾아, 각 그림의 상황에 맞는 대화를 완성하세요.

> 보기
> You had better take your pills three times a day.
> If you have to cough, hold a pillow against your stomach.
> Don't take long steps.

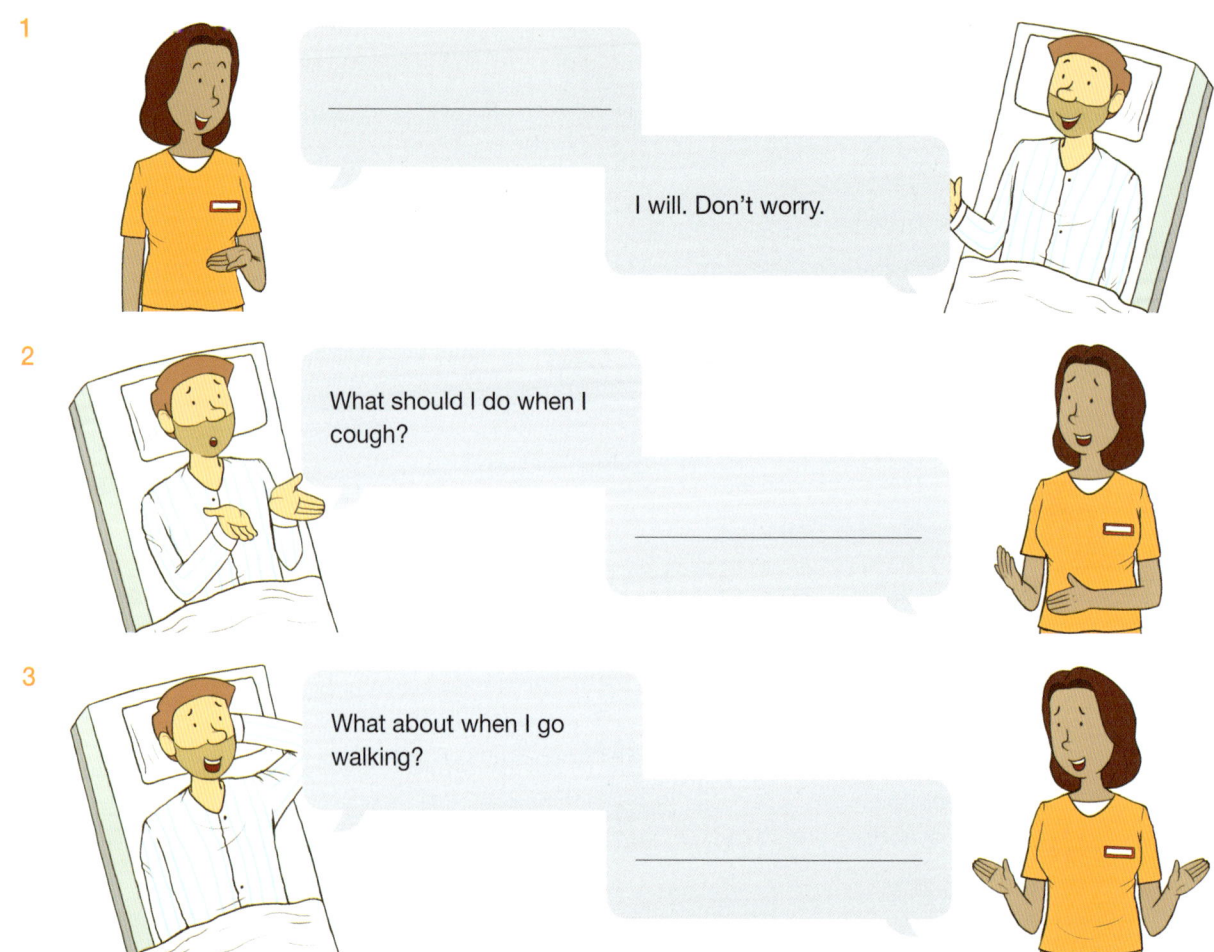

B 주어진 세 가지 상황을 이용하여, 파트너와 함께 각 상황에 맞는 대화를 연습해 보세요.

Situation	(a)	(b)	(c)
1	in the morning, afternoon, and evening	When you go to the bathroom	about walking
2	three times each day	If you laugh or cough	when you are walking
3	twice a day	Before you cough	when walking

Nurse   Be sure to take your medication (a)_____. Do that thirty minutes after you eat.

Patient   All right. I'll definitely take it every day.

Nurse   (b)_____, press a pillow against your abdomen. That will help ease the pain.

Patient   What about walking?

Nurse   Be careful (c)_____. Don't take long strides. Instead, take short steps.

Job Simulation II

A 〈보기〉에서 적절한 말을 찾아, 각 그림의 상황에 맞는 대화를 완성하세요.

> 보기
> It's covering half of the cost.
> How are you going to pay today?
> We have a copy of it in our records.

1

Should I give you my insurance card?

_____

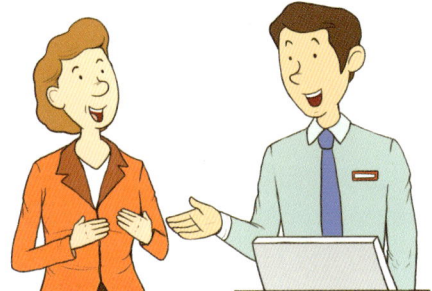

2

How much is my insurance paying today?

_____

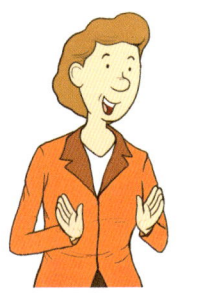

3

_____

I'm going to pay with cash.

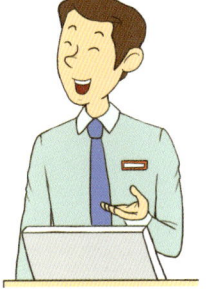

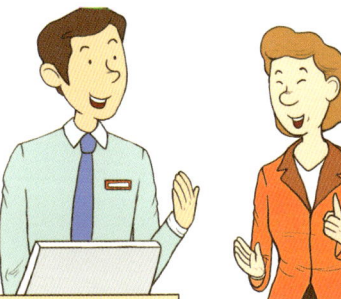

B 주어진 세 가지 상황을 이용하여, 파트너와 함께 각 상황에 맞는 대화를 연습해 보세요.

Situation	(a)	(b)	(c)
1	does my insurance cover	paying for half the cost	any cash
2	is my insurance company paying	covering 55% of everything	any cash on hand
3	does my medical insurance cover	taking care of 80% of this visit	enough money

Patient How much (a)_____ for this visit?

Receptionist Your insurance is (b)_____. You are responsible for the rest. How would you like to pay for that?

Patient I don't have (c)_____, so can I use a credit card?

Receptionist Yes, you can.

Reading & Listening

다음 지문을 읽고, 음성을 들어 보세요.

The Importance of Discharge Planning

Track 66

When doctors decide patients don't need to stay in the hospital any longer, they discharge them. However, most patients are not completely recovered yet. They must get better on their own at home. Therefore, discharge planning is very important. Nurses usually handle this. They must evaluate their patients' conditions, determine [1]what care or rehabilitation they need, provide referrals to other medical facilities or rehab centers, and arrange for follow-up appointments and tests. They should also provide their patients with prescriptions for medicine and [2]let them know how to take it. Before their patients are discharged, nurses must discuss all aspects of their continuing care. Patients often ask questions, so nurses should be prepared to answer them. Good discharge planning will ensure that patients recover quickly. It will also help them avoid relapses, so they won't have to be readmitted to the hospital.

Words & Phrases

discharge to send an inpatient home from the hospital
rehabilitation recovery from an illness, surgery, or injury that a person must do   **referral** a written recommendation that a patient visit another doctor or hospital   **relapse** the reoccurring of an injury or illness   **be readmitted** to be brought back to the hospital for something that had been treated before

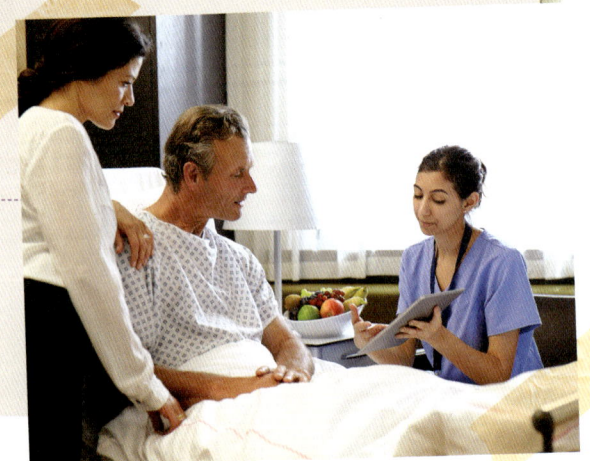

Basic Grammar

① 의문형용사 what

의문사 what이 뒤에 나오는 명사를 수식하는 형용사적 용법으로 쓰일 때는 '어떤', '무슨'이라는 의미를 나타낸다.

The doctor explained what treatment she would need.   의사는 그녀에게 어떤 치료가 필요할지 설명했다.
You can just choose what day you would like to visit.   무슨 요일에 방문하시고 싶은지 정하시면 됩니다.

② 사역동사 let

let은 '~하게 하다'라는 뜻으로, 본문에서는 '알다'라는 뜻의 동사원형 know를 목적격 보어로 취하여 '알게 하다'라는 뜻을 나타냈다.

They let the other nurses know their schedules for the month.   그들은 다른 간호사들에게 이달의 일정을 알려 주었다.
Dr. Min usually lets her patients decide what anesthesia they want.   민 선생님은 보통 환자들이 어떤 마취를 원하는지 결정하게 한다.

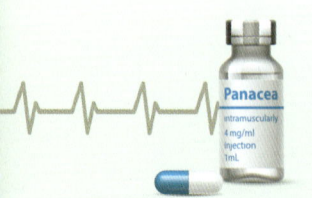

TIPS & TIPS

지금 만나러 갑니다.

간호사라고 해서 모두 병원에서만 근무하지는 않습니다. 가정간호사는 환자가 있는 가정에 직접 방문하여 환자를 돌보는 간호사를 말합니다. 이들은 간호 서비스를 제공할 뿐만 아니라, 환자가 식사를 하거나 씻는 것을 돕고, 옷을 갈아 입혀 주는 등 여러모로 환자에게 손과 발이 되어 줍니다. 가정간호사 서비스를 이용하는 환자는 다양한데요. 퇴원 후 집에서 회복을 기다리는 이들, 병에 걸리지는 않았지만 거동이 불편해서 일상 생활에 도움이 필요한 노인들, 그리고 난치병에 걸려 남은 생을 집에서 보내고자 하는 환자들입니다. 이들은 병원에 입원해 있지는 않지만 간호 서비스가 필요합니다. 바로 이런 사람들을 위해 가정간호사가 있는 것이지요.

UNIT 12
Handling Calls from Discharged Patients

Warmup
다음은 퇴원 후 어떤 증상이 있어, 병원에 전화한 환자들의 모습입니다. 각 환자와 문의 전화 내용을 연결해 보세요.

1.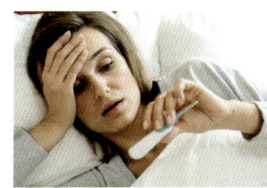

    a. "I have a fever. Do I need to go to the hospital?"

2.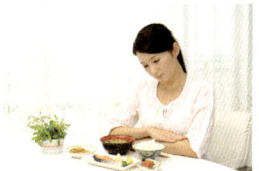

    b. "I am throwing up a lot."

3.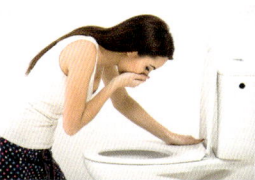

    c. "I have no appetite. Is this happening because of the medicine?"

Vocabulary
주어진 의미에 어울리는 단어를 고르세요.

1. prescription   • a. correctly
2. minor   • b. to say that something is bothering one
3. treat   • c. to care for; to take care of
4. complain   • d. directions for a pharmacist to provide a person with medication
5. properly   • e. small

Warmup Listening
Track 67
문장을 듣고 그에 맞는 대답을 고르세요.

1.
   a. Where are you?   b. Why not?
2.
   a. Let me ask the doctor.   b. Here is your medicine.
3.
   a. Yes, I have some pills.   b. Yes, but they aren't helping.

Conversation I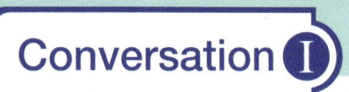

다음 대화를 듣고, 파트너와 함께 대화를 연습해 보세요.

Calls from Patients Who Need Something

Track 68

Nurse	Hello. Central Hospital. Dayoung speaking. How may I help you?
Patient	Hi. This is Jim Simmons. ¹Dr. Lee performed an operation on me last week. I was discharged from the hospital last week.
Nurse	Hello, Mr. Simmons. What can I do for you?
Patient	I have a small problem. I don't have enough medicine.
Nurse	²Why don't you have enough medicine? Dr. Lee gave you a prescription for two weeks' worth of medicine.
Patient	I'm really sorry, but I lost my medicine bottle. ³Do you think that I can get another prescription?
Nurse	For another prescription, you have to see the doctor again. Do you want to make an appointment to see Dr. Lee in the outpatient clinic?
Patient	Yes.

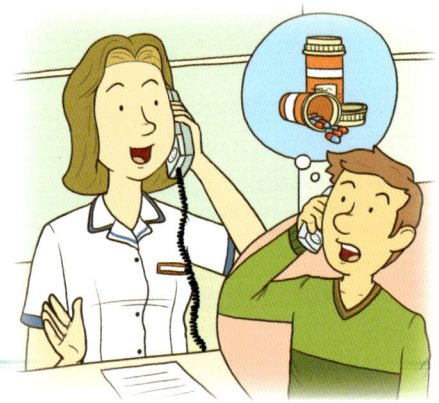

» Key Expressions

❶ Dr. Lee performed an operation on me last week.   이 선생님께서 지난주에 제 수술을 해 주셨어요.

환자가 어떤 의사에게 수술을 받았는지 나타내는 표현으로, 전치사 on 다음에 수술을 받은 당사자를 넣을 수 있다.

Dr. Hugh did an operation on my mother a week ago.   Hugh 선생님께서 일주일 전에 저희 어머니 수술을 해 주셨습니다.
I had an operation last Wednesday. My surgeon was Dr. Rolf.   저는 지난 수요일에 수술을 받았고요. 제 담당 의사는 Rolf 선생님이었어요.

❷ Why don't you have enough medicine?   왜 약이 충분하지 않으시지요?

환자에게 왜 처방약이 모자라는지 묻는 표현이다. why뿐만 아니라 how come도 '왜', '어째서'라는 의미로 사용할 수 있다.

Why is that?   왜 그렇지요?
How come you don't have enough medicine?   어째서 약이 충분하지 않으시지요?

❸ Do you think that I can get another prescription?   처방전을 하나 더 받을 수 있을까요?

환자가 처방전을 다시 받을 수 있는지 묻는 표현이다.

May I get another prescription?   처방전을 하나 더 받을 수 있을까요?
Is it possible for me to get another prescription?   처방전을 하나 더 받는 게 가능한가요?

Useful Phrases ➕

You can get ~   ~을 받으실 수 있습니다.

You can get another prescription. 처방전을 하나 더 받으실 수 있습니다.
You can get some pain medication anytime you want it. 원하실 때 언제든지 진통제를 받으실 수 있습니다.
You can get a test to see if you are immune to hepatitis B. 비형간염에 면역성이 있는지 확인하기 위해 검사를 받으실 수 있습니다.
You can get a referral to a physical therapist. 물리치료사 소개를 받으실 수 있습니다.

Basic Drills

A 주어진 문장에 어울리는 대답을 고르세요.

1. What can I do for you?
2. Why don't you have enough medicine?
3. Do you think that I can get another prescription?

a. I don't have enough medicine.
b. I lost my medicine bottle.
c. For another prescription, you have to see the doctor again.

B 괄호 안의 말을 순서대로 배열하여, 주어진 의미를 영어로 표현하세요.

1. 이 선생님께서 지난주에 제 수술을 해 주셨어요. (an operation / Dr. Lee / on me / performed / last week)

   _____

2. 왜 약이 충분하지 않으시지요? (have / don't you / medicine / why / enough)

   _____

3. 처방전을 하나 더 받을 수 있을까요? (I can / think that / do you / another / get / prescription)

   _____

Buildup Activities

대화를 듣고 빈칸을 채운 후, 주어진 질문에 답하세요.

Nurse   Hello. Dr. Chapman's office. This is Stephanie. Can I help you?

Patient   Hello. This is Paul Dawson. Dr. Chapman (a)_____ on me two weeks ago. I was (b)_____ from the hospital on Monday.

Nurse   Hello, Mr. Dawson. Is there something I can do for you?

Patient   Yes, there is. I have a problem. I'm (c)_____.

Nurse   Why don't you have any medicine? Dr. Chapman (d)_____ enough medicine for you for ten days.

Patient   I'm so sorry, but I left my medicine (e)_____. Would it be possible to get a new prescription?

Nurse   You need to see the doctor again to get another prescription. How about making an appointment to see him in the (f)_____ clinic?

Patient   That's fine.

1. What happened to the patient's medicine?
   a. He took all of it.
   b. He left it on the bus.
   c. He lost it at his home.

2. What will the nurse do next?
   a. talk to the doctor
   b. make a reservation
   c. see the patient

Conversation II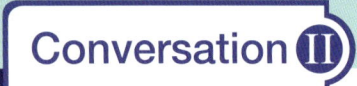

다음 대화를 듣고, 파트너와 함께 대화를 연습해 보세요.

Calls from Patients Who Are Complaining about Their Symptoms

Track 70

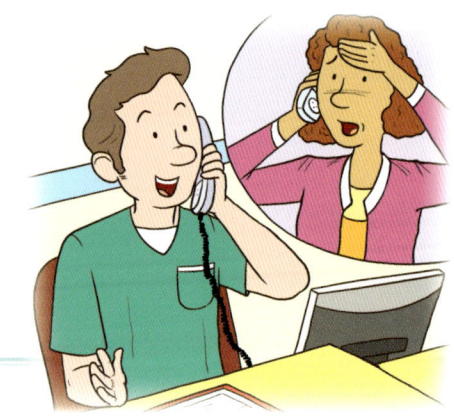

Nurse   Good morning. This is Dr. Simpson's office. How may I be of assistance?
Patient Hello. My name is Mary Nelson. Dr. Simpson treated me a couple of days ago.
Nurse   Yes, Ms. Nelson. ¹Do you need to see Dr. Simpson again?
Patient No, but ²I have a minor problem. I've had a bad headache since yesterday evening. And I have a bit of a fever.
Nurse   Have you been taking your medicine?
Patient Yes, I have, but I don't think it's working properly. ³I wonder if I can get a prescription for some new medicine.
Nurse   Let me talk to Dr. Simpson. He may need to see you again. Can I call you back in a few minutes?
Patient That would be great. Thanks. Goodbye.

» Key Expressions

❶ Do you need to see Dr. Simpson again?   Simpson 선생님께 다시 진료받으셔야 하나요?

퇴원 후 병원에 전화한 환자에게, 다시 내원해야 해서 전화했는지 묻는 표현이다.

Do you need to make another appointment with Dr. Bae?   배 선생님과 또 진료 약속을 잡으셔야 하나요?
Has something happened?   무슨 일 있으세요?

❷ I have a minor problem.   작은 문제가 하나 있어서요.

환자에게 작은 문제가 있다는 표현이다. minor(사소한)와 같이 문제의 심각성 정도를 나타낼 수 있는 형용사로는 small(작은), slight(가벼운), big(큰), serious(심각한) 등이 있다.

I have a serious matter to discuss with him. I can't move my legs.   선생님과 상의해야 할 심각한 문제가 있어요. 다리가 안 움직여요.

❸ I wonder if I can get a prescription for some new medicine.   새로운 약의 처방전을 받을 수 있는지 궁금합니다.

I wonder if ~(~인지 궁금합니다)를 사용하여 환자가 새로운 약의 처방전을 받을 수 있는지 묻고 있다. Do you think that ~?도 무엇이 가능한지 물어 볼 때 사용할 수 있다.

Do you think that you can give me something else?   저에게 다른 것을 주실 수 있을까요?
Is there any other medicine that I can take?   제가 먹을 수 있는 다른 약이 있나요?

Useful Phrases ➕

Have you been -ing? ~하고 있나요?

Have you been taking your medicine? 약은 드시고 있나요?
Have you been losing weight recently? 최근에 몸무게가 줄고 있나요?
Have you been experiencing any stress lately? 최근에 스트레스를 받고 있나요?
Have you been working out regularly? 꾸준히 운동을 하고 있나요?

Basic Drills

A 주어진 문장에 어울리는 대답을 고르세요.

1. Do you need to see Dr. Simpson again?
2. I wonder if I can get a prescription for some new medicine.
3. Have you been taking your medicine?

a. Let me talk to Dr. Simpson.
b. Yes, I have.
c. No, but I have a minor problem.

B 괄호 안의 말을 순서대로 배열하여, 주어진 의미를 영어로 표현하세요.

1. Simpson 선생님께 다시 진료받으셔야 하나요? (Dr. Simpson / do you / see / need to / again)

2. 작은 문제가 하나 있어서요. (a / problem / have / minor / I)

3. 새로운 약의 처방전을 받을 수 있는지 궁금합니다. (a prescription / if / I wonder / for / I can get / some new medicine)

Buildup Activities

Track 71

대화를 듣고 빈칸을 채운 후, 주어진 질문에 답하세요.

Nurse	Good afternoon. Dr. Taylor's office. How may I help you?
Patient	Hello. My name is Molly Reed. I visited Dr. Taylor (a)_____ days ago.
Nurse	Yes, Ms. Reed. Do you need to make another appointment with Dr. Taylor?
Patient	I don't think so, but I have a (b)_____. Since yesterday morning, I've had a terrible headache. I've also got a really (c)_____.
Nurse	Are you taking your (d)_____?
Patient	Yes, I am, but I don't think it's helping. Do you think Dr. Taylor can give me something (e)_____?
Nurse	I have to talk to Dr. Taylor first. He might want you to (f)_____ the office. Is it okay if I call you back in ten minutes?
Patient	That's fine. Thank you. Goodbye.
Nurse	Goodbye.

1. When did the patient see Dr. Taylor?
   a. yesterday   b. two days ago   c. three days ago

2. What does the patient request?
   a. another appointment   b. X-rays   c. some new medicine

Job Simulation I

A 〈보기〉에서 적절한 말을 찾아, 각 그림의 상황에 맞는 대화를 완성하세요.

> 보기
> Do you think I can get a new prescription?
> Why don't you have any medicine?
> Dr. Morrison performed surgery on me five days ago.

1 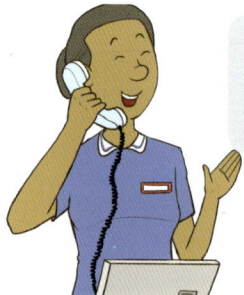 Can I help you? _____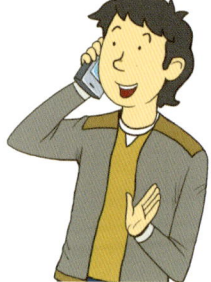

2 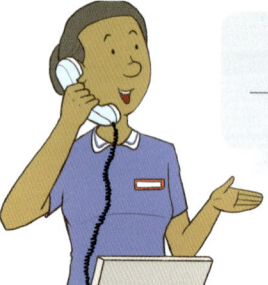 _____ I lost my medicine at work.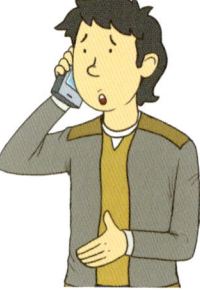

3 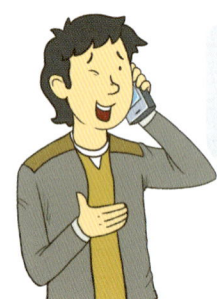 _____ You have to see the doctor again to get a new prescription.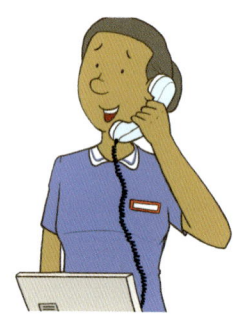

B 주어진 세 가지 상황을 이용하여, 파트너와 함께 각 상황에 맞는 대화를 연습해 보세요.

Situation	(a)	(b)
1	What happened to all of the medicine you had	have to come here to see the doctor
2	Where did all of your medicine go	must visit the doctor in person
3	Why have you already run out of medicine	need to schedule an appointment with the doctor

Nurse   (a)_____? Dr. Lee gave you a prescription for two weeks' worth of medicine.

Patient   I'm really sorry, but I lost my medicine bottle. Do you think that I can get another prescription?

Nurse   For another prescription, you (b)_____.

Job Simulation II

A 〈보기〉에서 적절한 말을 찾아, 각 그림의 상황에 맞는 대화를 완성하세요.

> 보기
> Yes, I am, but it's not helping me.
> No, but I have a small problem that I need to mention to you.
> I wonder if I can get a prescription for something else.

1 Do you want to see the doctor again?

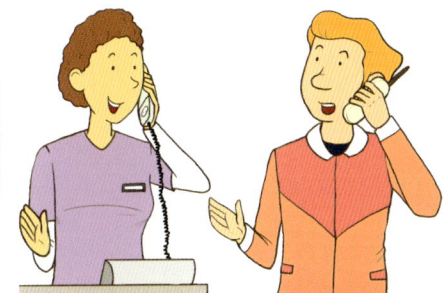

_____

2 Are you still taking your medicine?

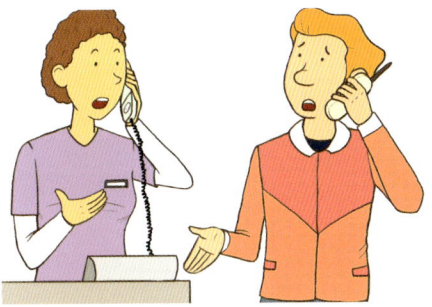

_____

3 _____

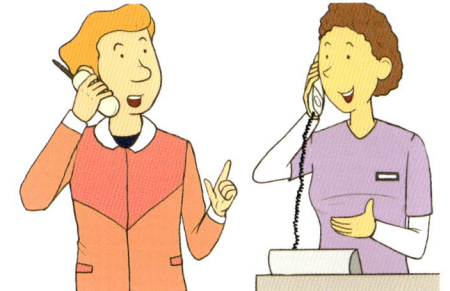

Let me discuss the matter with Dr. Thomas.

B 주어진 세 가지 상황을 이용하여, 파트너와 함께 각 상황에 맞는 대화를 연습해 보세요.

Situation	(a)	(b)	(c)
1	There is something wrong	taking your pills	some new medicine
2	I have a problem	taking your medicine three times a day	something else
3	I have an issue	following the directions regarding your medication	some medicine that is a bit stronger

Patient   (a)_____. I've had a bad headache since yesterday evening.

Nurse   Have you been (b)_____?

Patient   Yes, I have, but I don't think it's working properly. I wonder if I can get (c)_____.

Nurse   Let me talk to Dr. Simpson. Can I call you back in a few minutes?

Unit 12 | 105

Reading & Listening

다음 지문을 읽고, 음성을 들어 보세요.

What Is Medical Tourism?

Track 72

Most people travel to foreign countries to go sightseeing. But nowadays, some people [1]are traveling for medical reasons. Medical tourism is popular in countries such as India and Thailand. People visit those countries and others to [2]have medical procedures done. They engage in medical tourism for many reasons. One is price. The cost of some surgeries in India, Thailand, and other countries can be 90% cheaper than in the United States or European countries. There are very short waiting lists, too. Medical tourists get treated at hospitals with world-class facilities. The doctors at the hospitals speak English and other foreign languages. And they often studied at the world's top medical schools. In addition, some procedures may be illegal in the medical tourists' home countries but are allowed in other countries. Some countries make large amounts of money from medical tourism. So they are encouraging even more people to visit them for medical reasons.

Words & Phrases

engage in to take part in; to participate　**waiting list** a list of people waiting to do something　**world-class** outstanding; excellent　**top** best; highest　**illegal** not allowed by law; against the law

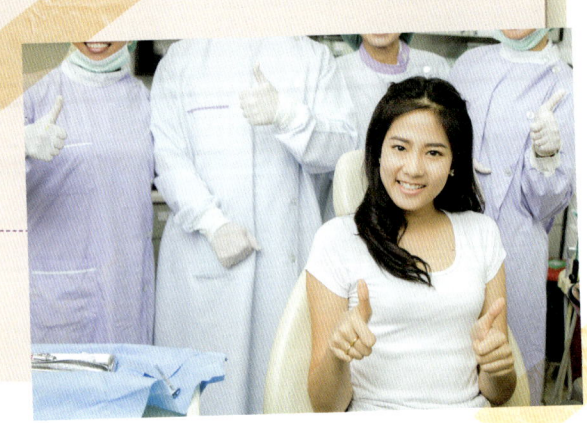

Basic Grammar

❶ 현재 진행형

현재 진행형은 be동사 + -ing의 형태를 취하며, 어떤 행동이 현재 진행 중임을 나타낸다. 하지만 '바로 지금 이 시각에' 진행 중이라는 의미뿐만 아니라, '최근에'와 같이 넓은 의미를 나타낼 수도 있다.

The patient is eating his breakfast.　환자가 아침 식사를 하고 있다.
Dr. Lloyd is treating him these days.　요즈음에는 Lloyd 의사가 그를 치료하고 있다.

❷ have + 목적어 + p.p.　목적어가 ~되도록 하다

5형식 사역동사 have를 사용하여, '목적어가 ~되도록 하다'라는 의미를 나타낸다. 과거분사(p.p.)는 수동의 의미이다.

I will have your bandage changed soon.　붕대가 곧 교체되도록 해 드리겠습니다.
Please call this number to have your medicine refilled.　약이 보충되도록 하시려면 이 번호로 전화해 주세요.

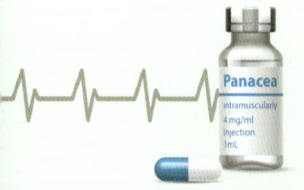

의료 관광, 안전한가요?

의료 관광이 주는 이점은 상당합니다. 하지만 그에 따르는 위험성도 무시할 수 없는데요. 먼저 환자의 상태에 따라 해외까지 이동하는 것이 무리일 수 있습니다. 외국에 있는 병원에 무사히 도착한다고 해도, 다른 문제에 맞닥뜨릴지도 모릅니다. 예를 들어, 위생 관리가 제대로 이루어지지 않는 병원이라면 일회용 주사기 등을 재사용하지 않는다는 보장이 없지요. 게다가 환자의 나라에는 없는 질병이나 바이러스에 노출될 수도 있고요. 혈액 안전 관리를 소홀히 하는 병원에 갔다가는 감염된 혈액을 공급받을 수도 있습니다. 이러한 의료 문제 말고도 언어의 장벽 때문에 의사소통이 힘들 수 있으며, 의료 과실 문제가 발생했을 때 소송 절차가 매우 까다롭거나 소송 자체가 불가능할 수도 있습니다.

Answer Key

Answer Key

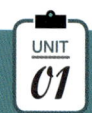 **Taking Reservations on the Phone**

Warmup p.11
1. c
2. b
3. a
4. d

Vocabulary
1. c
2. a
3. d
4. e
5. b

Warmup Listening
1. a
2. b
3. b

script Track 01

1. What would you like to see him for?
2. What about this Friday at one in the afternoon?
3. Would you like to reschedule your appointment?

Conversation I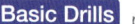

Basic Drills p.13
Ⓐ 1. c
2. b
3. a

Ⓑ 1. How may I help you?
2. What would you like to see him for?
3. What about this Friday at one in the afternoon?

Buildup Activities
script Track 03

Receptionist: Good morning. Central Hospital. How may I be of (a)assistance?

Patient: Hello. I want to make (b)an appointment to see Dr. Hamilton.

Receptionist: Why do you need to see her?

Patient: I don't (c)feel well these days. Are there any available times today?

Receptionist: Yes, there are. What about today at (d)eleven in the morning? Dr. Hamilton has time then.

Patient: I'm sorry, but that's a bad time for me. Do you have anything available sometime in (e)the afternoon?

Receptionist: Just a minute while I check . . . Ah, yes. How about this afternoon at (f)four fifteen?

Patient: That would be great. I'll go there at that time. My name is Roger Martin. I'm one of Dr. Hamilton's patients.

Receptionist: Okay, Mr. Martin. See you later today.

1. a
2. c

Conversation II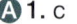

Basic Drills p.15
Ⓐ 1. c
2. a
3. b

Ⓑ 1. Are you calling to confirm your appointment?
2. Would you like to reschedule your appointment?
3. He has an appointment then, but he doesn't have anything scheduled for eight thirty.

Buildup Activities
script Track 05

Receptionist: Dr. Lee's office. Is there something I can help you with?

Patient: Hello. My name is Amy Butler. I am (a)supposed to see Dr. Lee at three o'clock this afternoon.

Receptionist: That's right, Ms. Butler. Do you need to see Dr. Lee before then?

Patient: No, I don't. In fact, I can't meet her today. I have to go (b)out of town right now.

Receptionist: I see. When is a (c)good time for you to see the doctor?

Patient: How about tomorrow morning (d)at nine?

Receptionist: Dr. Lee won't be here in the morning, but she will be here in the evening. (e)What about five forty-five?

Patient: That's kind of (f)late, but I have time then. Thanks for your help.

Receptionist: It's my pleasure. Have a nice day.

108

1. b 2. c

Job Simulation I p.16

A 1. I'd like to schedule an appointment with Dr. Min.
2. Why do you need to see the doctor?
3. How does this Thursday at two thirty sound to you?

Job Simulation II p.17

A 1. Did you call to confirm your appointment?
2. Do you want to reschedule your appointment for another day?
3. He's occupied then, but he's got an open slot at two fifteen.

UNIT 02 Receiving Patients

Warmup p.19

1. head
2. eye
3. nose
4. ear
5. neck
6. shoulder
7. chest
8. arm
9. waist
10. stomach
11. leg
12. foot

Vocabulary

1. a
2. c
3. e
4. b
5. d

Warmup Listening

1. b 2. a 3. a

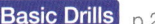

script

1. Is this your first time at this hospital?
2. How about filling out all of these forms?
3. How long have you had these symptoms?

Conversation I

Basic Drills p.21

A 1. a 2. c 3. b

B 1. Is this your first time to visit Dr. Kang?
2. It should take about ten minutes.
3. Why don't you complete the forms and bring them back when you're finished?

Buildup Activities

script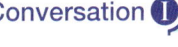

Patient: Hello. My name is Deanna Carpenter. I'm (a)scheduled to see Dr. Simmons at ten thirty.

Receptionist: Good morning, Ms. Carpenter. Have you seen Dr. Simmons before?

Patient: No, I haven't. This is my (b)first time to visit his office.

Receptionist: All right. Would you please (c)fill out these forms then? It will take around fifteen minutes.

Patient: Sure. I can do that.

Receptionist: And I need to see your (d)insurance card if you have it.

Patient: This is my (e)card.

Receptionist: Thank you very much. How about (f)completing all of the forms? Then, bring them back when you're done.

Patient: Okay. I'll be back in a bit.

1. a 2. b

Conversation II

Basic Drills p.23

A 1. b 2. a 3. c

B 1. Does your head hurt?
2. How long have you had these symptoms?
3. Let me check your temperature and pulse.

Buildup Activities

script

Nurse: Hello, Mr. Thompson. What's the matter with you today?

Patient: I feel like I'm coming down with (a)<u>a cold</u>. I feel awful right now.

Nurse: That's bad news. What (b)<u>symptoms</u> do you have?

Patient: My (c)<u>throat hurts</u>, and I've got a runny nose. My ears won't pop either. Lastly, I've got a slight fever.

Nurse: Do you have any aches and pains? Are you getting any (d)<u>headaches</u>?

Patient: No, my head and the rest of my body are fine.

Nurse: Okay, that doesn't seem bad. When did these symptoms start?

Patient: I began feeling bad yesterday afternoon while I was (e)<u>at work</u>.

Nurse: All right. I need to check your (f)<u>temperature</u> and pulse . . . Dr. Kim will be here to see you in just a moment.

1. c   2. c

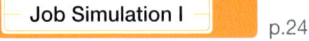

A 1. Yes, I am. I'm a new patient.

    2. May I see your insurance card?

    3. All right. I'll be back in a few minutes.

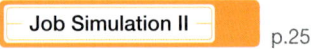

A 1. For instance, do you have a headache?

    2. I started to get sick this morning.

    3. I have to check your temperature and pulse.

UNIT 03 — Checking the Conditions of Patients

Warmup p.27

1. mild   2. moderate   3. severe

Vocabulary

1. e   2. d   3. b
4. a   5. c

Warmup Listening

1. b   2. a   3. b

script

1. It looks like you've gained some weight recently.
2. Is this pain constant?
3. When did the pain start?

Conversation I

Basic Drills p.29

A 1. b   2. c   3. a

B 1. Please roll up your sleeve and put your arm into the machine.

    2. Please step on the scale.

    3. How many bowel movements do you have a day?

Buildup Activities

script

Nurse: I need to check your (a)<u>blood pressure</u>. Would you please roll up your sleeve and put your arm into the machine?

Patient: All right. Do you want me to press the button?

Nurse: Yes, please . . . Okay, your blood pressure is 130 over 90. That's (b)<u>a little high</u>. Next, how about stepping on the scale?

Patient: No problem . . . I'm (c)<u>65</u> kilograms.

Nurse: It looks like you've (d)<u>lost</u> some weight recently. And how many (e)<u>bowel movements</u> do you have each day?

110

Patient: 1 or 2. But I've already had to visit the bathroom (f)<u>5 times</u> this morning.

Nurse: Are they watery?

Patient: No, they look good.

1. c   2. c

Conversation II

Basic Drills p.31

A 1. a   2. c   3. b

B 1. Is the pain constant, or does it come and go?

2. It's very sharp, and it won't go away.

3. The doctor will be here soon to examine you.

Buildup Activities

script   Track 17

Nurse: What brings you to the hospital today?

Patient: My (a)<u>stomach</u> really hurts.

Nurse: Can you tell me where it hurts?

Patient: Hmm . . . It mostly hurts in my (b)<u>lower</u> stomach. It also hurts a bit on the left side of my upper stomach.

Nurse: I see. Does it feel (c)<u>the same</u> all the time?

Patient: No, it's not constant. It's a (d)<u>stabbing</u> pain, and it sometimes goes away.

Nurse: When did you feel the pain first?

Patient: Around noon. It wasn't that painful at first, but it has been (e)<u>very severe</u> since three o'clock. Do you think this is serious?

Nurse: I can't tell. The doctor will be here to (f)<u>examine</u> you in a moment.

1. a   2. b

Job Simulation I p.32

A 1. Can you roll up your sleeve and put your arm into the machine, please?

2. Your blood pressure is 140 over 90.

3. Around 1 or 2 normally.

Job Simulation II p.33

A 1. Yes, the pain is constant.

2. It's a dull pain that won't go away.

3. I can't tell. Dr. Wilson will be with you in one moment.

UNIT 04 Giving Directions in and out of Buildings

Warmup p.35

1. b   2. c
3. d   4. a

Vocabulary

1. a   2. c   3. d
4. e   5. b

Warmup Listening

1. b   2. b   3. a

script   Track 19

1. I don't know where to go.

2. Can you tell me his name, please?

3. How do I get there?

Conversation I

Basic Drills p.37

A 1. c   2. b   3. a

B 1. The Cardiology Department is located on the fifth floor.

2. Do you see the elevators over there by the nurses' station?

3. When you get off the elevator, turn left and walk straight down the hall.

Buildup Activities
script Track 21

Patient: Pardon me, but could you give me (a)<u>a hand</u>, please?

Receptionist: I'll do my best. What do you need, ma'am?

Patient: I'm trying to find the maternity (b)<u>ward</u>. I am scheduled to meet Dr. Jeon in a few minutes, but I can't find my way there.

Receptionist: The maternity ward is on the (c)<u>third floor</u>.

Patient: Can you tell me how I can get up there?

Receptionist: Sure. Do you see the (d)<u>escalator</u> over there by the ATM?

Patient: Yes, I see it.

Receptionist: Take it up to the third floor. Get off the escalator and (e)<u>walk straight</u> to the end of the hall. The maternity ward will be (f)<u>on your left</u>.

Patient: Thank you very much. You've been quite helpful.

1. c   2. b

Conversation II

Basic Drills p.39

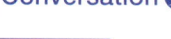 1. a   2. b   3. c

 1. How do you spell her last name?
2. Your sister is in room 322 in Building B.
3. Walk straight that way and go out the back door.

Buildup Activities
script Track 23

Visitor: Good evening. (a)<u>My aunt</u> is hospitalized here, so I'm visiting her. Could you please tell me what room she is in?

Receptionist: I sure can. What's her (b)<u>name</u>?

Visitor: It's Amelia Smith.

Receptionist: How do you (c)<u>spell</u> her first name?

Visitor: It's A-M-E-L-I-A.

Receptionist: Aha, here she is. You can find her in room 503 in (d)<u>Building 3</u>. In case you don't know, we're in Building 1.

Visitor: Oh, she's in another building. Where is it?

Receptionist: Walk out the (e)<u>side door</u> of this building. After that, take a left. You'll see a very tall white building. That's Building 3. Go right into it through the front doors and take the elevator to the (f)<u>fifth floor</u>. A nurse can help you if you can't find your way.

Visitor: Thanks for all your help. I appreciate it.

1. b   2. c

Job Simulation I p.40

 1. I'm not sure where I should go.
2. Can you see the elevators next to the nurses' station?
3. When you get off the elevator, turn right and walk about 30 meters.

Job Simulation II p.41

 1. Can you please tell me her name?
2. Your mother is hospitalized in room 912 in Building 5.
3. Walk that way and head out the back door.

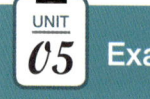
UNIT 05 Examinations I

Warmup p.43

1. take a seat
2. roll up one's sleeve
3. make a fist
4. lie down

Vocabulary

1. c   2. b   3. d

4. e   5. a

Warmup Listening

1. b   2. b   3. a

script   Track 25

1. I have to get a blood sample from you.
2. What do you need from me?
3. What should I do with this container?

Conversation I

Basic Drills p.45

Ⓐ 1. c   2. b   3. a

Ⓑ 1. I'll draw some blood from you.
2. Please make a fist with your left hand and just relax.
3. You might feel a little sting.

Buildup Activities

script   Track 27

Nurse: The doctor asked me to run some (a)blood tests on you today. So I have to take some blood.

Patient: Will this hurt? I don't like (b)needles very much.

Nurse: You don't need to worry at all. Would you please sit down and (c)hold out your right arm?

Patient: No problem. What do you want me to do next?

Nurse: Make a fist with your right hand. Then, just sit back and relax. You can close your eyes if you want. You'll barely feel anything . . . All right. I'm all finished. I'll put this (d)bandage on your arm. Do you feel all right?

Patient: No, I don't. I feel a little (e)lightheaded now.

Nurse: You'd better (f)lie down for a minute. You can lie down here. You'll be as good as new in no time.

Patient: Thanks.

1. a   2. b

Conversation II

Basic Drills p.47

Ⓐ 1. c   2. a   3. b

Ⓑ 1. We need a urine sample and a stool sample.
2. Please get some urine in this container and stool in the other one.
3. Make sure the labels on the containers are facing outward.

Buildup Activities

script   Track 29

Nurse: Dr. Yoon doesn't know what's wrong with you yet. So we have to run a few tests. We have to get a urine sample and a (a)stool sample from you.

Patient: I just went to the bathroom ten minutes ago. I can't (b)urinate right now.

Nurse: That's fine. How about drinking (c)some water and waiting a few minutes then? . . . Okay, Mr. Simpson, are you ready? Take these two containers to the bathroom. Please urinate in this one and defecate in the other one. The bathroom is down the hall on the left.

Patient: Do you want me to bring the (d)containers back here?

Nurse: Please don't. There's a (e)cabinet in the bathroom. You can put the containers in it. Just be sure the (f)labels with your name on them are facing outward.

Patient: Okay. I'll be back here in a bit.

1. c   2. a

Job Simulation I p.48

Ⓐ 1. I need to get some blood from you.
2. Could you please make a fist with your left hand and relax?
3. This might sting a bit.

Job Simulation II p.49

Ⓐ 1. I don't think I can urinate right now.

2. You need to urinate in this container and defecate in the other.

3. Be sure that the labels on the containers are facing outward.

UNIT 06 Examinations II

Warmup p.51

hearing aid, glasses, necklace, false teeth, cell phone, watch, belt

Vocabulary

1. a 2. c 3. b
4. e 5. d

Warmup Listening

1. a 2. b 3. b

script Track 31

1. Do you have any jewelry on?
2. I need to rub this on your stomach.
3. Can you turn to the right?

Conversation I

Basic Drills p.53

Ⓐ 1. b 2. a 3. c

Ⓑ 1. Are you wearing any jewelry?
2. You need to remove the necklace.
3. You must remain still during the entire process.

Buildup Activities

script Track 33

Nurse: You're going to get an (a)MRI scan. Do you have any jewelry on? Are there any credit cards or (b)debit cards in your wallet?

Patient: Yes, there are a few cards. And I'm wearing a (c)bracelet as well.

Nurse: Please take off the bracelet and leave your wallet here, too. You can't have anything (d)metallic on you when you're in the machine. All right, it's very easy. Just lie down here.

Patient: What (e)position should I be in?

Nurse: Lie on your back. And please remain still the entire time. If you move, we'll have to do the exam over. The machine is noisy, but don't worry. This will last about (f)ten minutes. Shall we begin?

Patient: Let's do it.

1. c 2. b

Conversation II

Basic Drills p.55

Ⓐ 1. b 2. c 3. a

Ⓑ 1. She wants to know what is causing the swelling in your body.
2. I'm going to rub some jelly on your stomach.
3. Please turn to your left a bit.

Buildup Activities

script Track 35

Nurse: Mr. Jenkins, the doctor wants to do an (a)ultrasound scan on you. We need to look at the (b)swollen part of your body. Can you get onto the examination table, please?

Patient: All right.

Nurse: Please (c)pull up your shirt to expose your stomach and wait for a moment . . .

Doctor: I'm going to put some (d)jelly on your stomach. It's pretty cold.

Patient: Yeah, it is. What is the jelly for?

Doctor: It helps (e)transmit sound waves better, so it makes better images. Please don't move while I am using the transducer . . . All right, can you turn to the (f)right?

Patient: Like this?

Doctor: Yes, exactly.

1. b 2. a

114

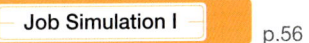 **Job Simulation I** p.56

Ⓐ 1. Are you wearing any kind of jewelry?
2. You need to remove the earrings and necklace.
3. You have to remain still during the entire process.

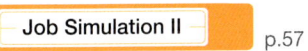 **Job Simulation II** p.57

Ⓐ 1. We have to figure out what is causing the swelling in your body.
2. I'm going to put some of this jelly on your stomach.
3. What is this jelly for?

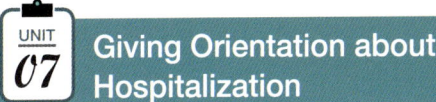
UNIT 07 Giving Orientation about Hospitalization

Warmup p.59

1. television 2. window
3. cabinet   4. chair
5. folding table 6. pillow
7. bedsheet   8. bedside table

Vocabulary

1. d   2. e   3. a
4. c   5. b

Warmup Listening

1. a   2. b   3. a

Track 37

script

1. What is this button for?
2. When are the hospital's visiting hours?
3. Can I get soy milk instead of regular milk?

Conversation Ⓘ

Basic Drills p.61

Ⓐ 1. c   2. b   3. a

Ⓑ 1. When you need help, just press the button.
2. We serve breakfast at 8 AM and lunch at noon.
3. The hospital's visiting hours are 10 AM to 8 PM on weekdays and 9 AM to 10 PM on weekends.

Buildup Activities

Track 39

script

Nurse: Here is your room, Mr. Emerson. You'll stay here until you (a)<u>recover</u>. There are your bed and bedside table.

Patient: What's (b)<u>this button</u>?

Nurse: It's the call button. Press that button if you need to see (c)<u>a nurse</u>. One of us will come here at once.

Patient: If I am (d)<u>in pain</u>, should I press it?

Nurse: Yes, you should. In addition, you'll eat three times each day. We serve breakfast at 7:30 and lunch at noon. Your dinner will arrive at 6:30.

Patient: What are the hospital's (e)<u>visiting hours</u>? My family is planning to visit me each day.

Nurse: (f)<u>On weekdays</u>, visiting hours run from 9 AM to 7 PM, and they last from 8 AM to 9 PM on weekends.

Patient: Thanks for your explanations.

1. b   2. a

Conversation Ⅱ

Basic Drills p.63

Ⓐ 1. b   2. a   3. c

Ⓑ 1. I'm very sorry, but we only provide those to patients.
2. Can I get soy milk instead of regular milk?
3. I'll talk to the dietician and see if that is okay.

Buildup Activities

Track 41

script

Patient: Pardon me, nurse, but I have a question. (a)<u>My son</u> wants to take a nap. Can you get a blanket and a pillow for him, please?

Answer Key | 115

Nurse: I'm terribly sorry, but we (b)only give those to patients. We can't let visitors have them.

Patient: That's fine. By the way, I have a question about my food.

Nurse: Sure. What is it?

Patient: Can I get (c)eggs instead of tofu? I don't really like tofu.

Nurse: Let me talk to the (d)dietician and see if that is okay. Are there any other questions?

Patient: Yes, I have one last question. Where can I get toiletries such as (e)soap and shampoo?

Nurse: There's a (f)convenience store on the first floor.

1. a   2. b

Job Simulation I   p.64

A 1. When you need assistance, just press it.
2. We serve breakfast at 8:30 and lunch at noon every day.
3. They last from 10 to 7 on weekdays and run from 9 to 8 on weekends.

Job Simulation II   p.65

A 1. I'm sorry, but we only let patients use them.
2. May I have soy milk instead of regular milk?
3. I'll speak to the dietician to see if that is possible.

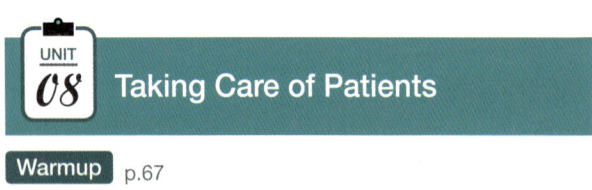

UNIT 08 — Taking Care of Patients

Warmup   p.67
2 – 3 – 1

Vocabulary
1. a   2. d   3. b
4. c   5. e

Warmup Listening
1. b   2. b   3. a

Track 43

script
1. How do you feel today?
2. This is starting to itch a lot.
3. Why do I have to change positions?

Conversation I

Basic Drills   p.69

A 1. a   2. c   3. b

B 1. I feel better today than I did yesterday.
2. It is really starting to itch a lot.
3. You appear to be improving rapidly.

Buildup Activities

script   Track 45

Nurse: Good morning, Mr. Pennington. How are you doing this morning?

Patient: I think I'm improving. I feel (a)a little better today than I did yesterday.

Nurse: That's great news. It's time for me to change your (b)dressing.

Patient: Good. It (c)itches a lot.

Nurse: Would you please lie down on the bed? Then, I can put a (d)new bandage on. That will make you stop itching.

Patient: Okay.

Nurse: Hmm . . . Your cut is (e)healing slowly, but it's not infected. You should start to (f)improve in a few days.

Patient: That's nice to know. Thank you.

1. c   2. a

Conversation II

Basic Drills   p.71

A 1. b   2. a   3. c

B 1. You ought to change your position every two hours when you are in bed.
   2. If you lie in the same position, it will decrease the blood flow to some parts of your body.
   3. You can develop bedsores.

Buildup Activities

script Track **47**

Nurse: Mr. Kimball, it's five o'clock. It's time to change (a)<u>positions</u>.

Patient: Didn't I do that a few hours ago?

Nurse: Yes, you did. But you're supposed to change positions every (b)<u>two hours</u> when you are in bed.

Patient: Really? (c)<u>Why</u> am I supposed to do that?

Nurse: Lying in the same position will (d)<u>decrease</u> the blood flowing to certain parts of your body. That will weaken the tissue in those places.

Patient: Is that a bad thing?

Nurse: Yes, it is. You might get (e)<u>bedsores</u>. Infected bedsores can cause serious problems. That's why patients need to rotate positions regularly.

Patient: I understand. I'll be sure to turn (f)<u>every two hours</u> in that case.

1. b   2. c

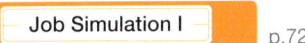 p.72

A 1. I feel a great deal better today.
   2. Excellent. It itches a lot.
   3. There is no sign of infection around your cut.

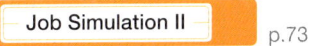 p.73

A 1. You need to change positions every two hours when you are in bed.
   2. Lying in the same position will decrease the blood flow to certain parts of your body.
   3. Okay. I'll be sure to rotate more often then.

 Discussing Medication

Warmup p.75

1. d   2. c
3. a   4. b

Vocabulary

1. d   2. e   3. a
4. b   5. c

Warmup Listening

1. a   2. a   3. b

script Track **49**

1. It's time for your medicine.
2. Does the medicine have any side effects?
3. What are these pills for?

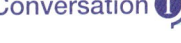

Basic Drills p.77

A 1. c   2. b   3. a

B 1. It's time for your medication.
   2. I'm going to put your medication into the IV drip.
   3. You might feel a bit nauseous, and you may develop a skin rash.

Buildup Activities

script Track **51**

Nurse: Good evening, Mr. Buford. I have to give you your (a)<u>medication</u> now.

Patient: Good evening. You're not going to give me a (b)<u>shot</u>, are you?

Nurse: No, I'm not. I've got some (c)<u>pills</u> for you to take.

Patient: Good. I don't like (d)<u>needles</u> very much.

Nurse: This medicine is going to make you feel a bit sleepy. In fact, you're probably going to take a nap soon.

Answer Key | 117

Patient: Does it have any other (e)side effects?

Nurse: You might get a bit dizzy, and you (f)may itch a bit. Please tell me if either of these happens to you. Then, the doctor can adjust your level of medication.

Patient: Okay, I'll do that. Wow, I am already getting sleepy. I think I'm going to fall asleep now.

1. c   2. a

Basic Drills p.79

Ⓐ 1. b   2. c   3. a

Ⓑ 1. These pills help prevent blood clots from forming.
 2. Patients who have heart surgery commonly get all of these types of medicine.
 3. Let me bring you a sheet of paper.

Buildup Activities

script   Track 53

Nurse: It's time for your medicine, Mr. Marino.

Patient: That's a lot (a)of pills. What are they all for?

Nurse: These pills will keep (b)blood clots from developing. This medication will help decrease your blood pressure. And this one is a pain reliever. It will stop your body from hurting so much.

Patient: Is it (c)safe to take so many pills at once?

Nurse: Yes, it is. Organ transplant patients usually get all of these kinds of medicine.

Patient: Is it okay to take them on an (d)empty stomach?

Nurse: Absolutely not. You shouldn't do that. They could give you a stomachache, make you feel (e)nauseous, or make you throw up.

Patient: What about the side effects of all this medicine?

Nurse: I will bring you a pamphlet in a minute. It (f)explains the side effects of each medicine you're taking.

1. b   2. c

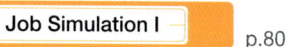

Ⓐ 1. It's time for you to take your medicine.
 2. I'm going to put your medication in your IV drip.
 3. You may feel nauseous or develop a rash on your skin.

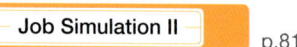

Ⓐ 1. These pills will help prevent your body from getting infected.
 2. Liver transplant patients usually have to take these.
 3. I'll bring you a sheet of paper that explains all of them.

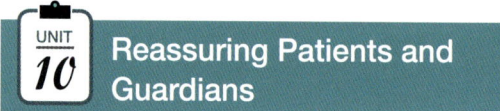

Warmup p.83

2 – 4 – 3 – 1

Vocabulary

1. b   2. d   3. e
4. c   5. a

Warmup Listening

1. a   2. b   3. a

script   Track 55

1. How do you feel?
2. Were there any complications?
3. Can I see my daughter?

Basic Drills p.85

Ⓐ 1. b   2. a   3. c

Ⓑ 1. Can you tell me your name?

118

2. How do you feel?

3. You feel that way because of the anesthesia.

Buildup Activities

script   Track 57

Patient: Oh . . . Where . . . Where am I?

Nurse: Ah, you're (a)<u>awake</u>. Do you know your name?

Patient: My name . . . ? Yeah, I'm Peter Robinson.

Nurse: Well done, Mr. Robinson.

Patient: Can you tell me (b)<u>where</u> I am?

Nurse: You're in the (c)<u>recovery room</u> at Central Hospital. Your operation went well. How are you feeling? Why don't you try to open your eyes?

Patient: I (d)<u>feel awful</u>. I want to open my eyes, but I can't.

Nurse: That will be hard to do for a while because of the anesthesia. Do you have any pain?

Patient: (e)<u>My head</u> hurts really badly. And my throat is dry. Can I get a drink of water?

Nurse: Not yet. You're not allowed to drink anything for (f)<u>another hour</u>.

1. b   2. c

Conversation II

Basic Drills p.87

Ⓐ 1. a   2. b   3. c

Ⓑ 1. Everything worked out fine.

2. She's still in the recovery room and hasn't woken up yet.

3. Why don't you sit down and relax?

Buildup Activities

script   Track 59

Guardian: How was Gina Gilman's (a)<u>operation</u>? Were there any problems?

Nurse: The operation was successful, sir. (b)<u>Your wife's</u> surgeon will speak with you about it in a moment.

Guardian: Can I (c)<u>visit</u> her now?

Nurse: She's still sleeping in the recovery room. You have to wait until she wakes up.

Guardian: When will she be (d)<u>awake</u>?

Nurse: She will probably wake up in about (e)<u>half an hour</u>. You can see her in her room in an hour or so.

Guardian: Okay. Thank you.

Nurse: How about (f)<u>sitting down</u> and relaxing a bit? Dr. Wilson will be here soon.

1. a   2. b

Job Simulation I   p.88

Ⓐ 1. Can you remember your name?

2. How do you feel?

3. The anesthesia is making you feel that way.

Job Simulation II   p.89

Ⓐ 1. The operation was 100% successful.

2. She's still sleeping in the recovery room.

3. How about sitting down and relaxing for a bit?

UNIT 11 Discharging Patients

Warmup p.91

ⓐ, ⓒ

Vocabulary

1. c   2. b   3. a

4. e   5. d

Warmup Listening

1. a   2. b   3. b

script Track 61

1. Take this medicine three times a day.
2. Do you need my insurance card?
3. How do you want to pay your bill?

Conversation I

Basic Drills p.93

A 1. c   2. a   3. b

B 1. Be sure to take your medication three times a day.
2. If you have to cough, press a pillow against your abdomen.
3. Don't take long strides.

Buildup Activities

script Track 63

Nurse: You're being (a)discharged today, Mr. Wake, but you still have several things to do at home.

Patient: Okay, what kinds of things?

Nurse: You have to take your medicine daily. Take it (b)two times a day after meals. Be sure you take all your pills.

Patient: Don't worry. I'll take all of (c)my medicine.

Nurse: Whenever you cough, hold (d)a pillow against your stomach. That will make you feel less pain.

Patient: What about when I (e)go walking?

Nurse: Be very careful. Don't walk fast. Instead, you should (f)walk slowly.

Patient: I'll be sure to remember that.

1. b   2. c

Conversation II

Basic Drills p.95

A 1. a   2. c   3. b

B 1. We already have that information in our records.
2. Your insurance is covering fifty percent of the cost.
3. How would you like to pay for that?

Buildup Activities

script Track 65

Receptionist: This is (a)your bill, Ms. Patterson.

Patient: Thank you. Would you like (b)to see my insurance card?

Receptionist: That's all right. We have your insurance (c)information on file already.

Patient: How much does my insurance pay this time?

Receptionist: It's covering (d)sixty percent of the cost. You have to pay the rest. How are you going to pay today?

Patient: I didn't go to (e)the ATM today, so I need to pay with a credit card.

Receptionist: That's fine.

Patient: Here it is.

Receptionist: Thank you . . . Sign here, please . . . And this is (f)your receipt.

1. c   2. a

Job Simulation I p.96

A 1. You had better take your pills three times a day.
2. If you have to cough, hold a pillow against your stomach.
3. Don't take long steps.

Job Simulation II p.97

A 1. We have a copy of it in our records.
2. It's covering half of the cost.
3. How are you going to pay today?

UNIT 12 Handling Calls from Discharged Patients

Warmup p.99

1. a   2. c   3. b

Vocabulary

1. d   2. e   3. c
4. b   5. a

Warmup Listening

1. b   2. a   3. b

script   Track 67

1. I don't have enough medicine.
2. Can I get a new prescription?
3. Have you been taking your pills?

Conversation I

Basic Drills p.101

A 1. a   2. b   3. c

B 1. Dr. Lee performed an operation on me last week.
2. Why don't you have enough medicine?
3. Do you think that I can get another prescription?

Buildup Activities

script   Track 69

Nurse: Hello. Dr. Chapman's office. This is Stephanie. Can I help you?

Patient: Hello. This is Paul Dawson. Dr. Chapman (a)<u>operated</u> on me two weeks ago. I was (b)<u>discharged</u> from the hospital on Monday.

Nurse: Hello, Mr. Dawson. Is there something I can do for you?

Patient: Yes, there is. I have a problem. I'm (c)<u>out of medicine</u>.

Nurse: Why don't you have any medicine? Dr. Chapman (d)<u>prescribed</u> enough medicine for you for ten days.

Patient: I'm so sorry, but I left my medicine (e)<u>on the bus</u>. Would it be possible to get a new prescription?

Nurse: You need to see the doctor again to get another prescription. How about making an appointment to see him in the (f)<u>outpatient</u> clinic?

Patient: That's fine.

1. b   2. b

Conversation II

Basic Drills p.103

A 1. c   2. a   3. b

B 1. Do you need to see Dr. Simpson again?
2. I have a minor problem.
3. I wonder if I can get a prescription for some new medicine.

Buildup Activities

script   Track 71

Nurse: Good afternoon. Dr. Taylor's office. How may I help you?

Patient: Hello. My name is Molly Reed. I visited Dr. Taylor (a)<u>three</u> days ago.

Nurse: Yes, Ms. Reed. Do you need to make another appointment with Dr. Taylor?

Patient: I don't think so, but I have a (b)<u>slight problem</u>. Since yesterday morning, I've had a terrible headache. I've also got a really (c)<u>sore throat</u>.

Nurse: Are you taking your (d)<u>medicine</u>?

Patient: Yes, I am, but I don't think it's helping. Do you think Dr. Taylor can give me something (e)<u>stronger</u>?

Nurse: I have to talk to Dr. Taylor first. He might want you to (f)<u>visit</u> the office. Is it okay if I call you back in ten minutes?

Patient: That's fine. Thank you. Goodbye.

Nurse: Goodbye.

1. c   2. c

Job Simulation I   p.104

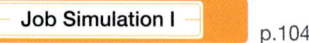 1. Dr. Morrison performed surgery on me five days ago.

2. Why don't you have any medicine?

3. Do you think I can get a new prescription?

Job Simulation II   p.105

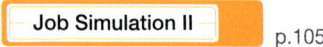 1. No, but I have a small problem that I need to mention to you.

2. Yes, I am, but it's not helping me.

3. I wonder if I can get a prescription for something else.

Appendix: Word List

Word List

Unit 01

appointment *n.* (진료) 예약, 약속
a scheduled meeting

annual *adj.* 매년의, 연례의
happening once a year; yearly

checkup *n.* 건강 검진
a general medical examination; a health exam

available *adj.* 이용할 수 있는
open; empty

hold on 기다리다
to wait

sound *v.* ~인 것 같다, ~처럼 들리다
to seem; to appear

reserve *v.* 예약하다
to book; to schedule a time and day to do something

patient *n.* 환자
a person who is being treated at a hospital

be of assistance 도움이 되다
to help

feel well 몸 상태가 좋다
to be healthy; to have no health problems

check *v.* 확인하다
to look for something

assist *v.* 돕다
to help

correct *adj.* 맞는, 정확한
right

confirm *v.* 확인하다, 확증하다
to make sure that something is right

client *n.* 고객, 의뢰인
a customer

reschedule *v.* 일정을 변경하다
to change the time or day of an appointment

early *adj.* 이른
happening before an expected time

make it (어떤 곳에) 시간 맞춰 가다
to go to a place

assistance *n.* 도움, 원조
help

go out of ~를 떠나다
to leave; to exit

Unit 02

fill out ~을 작성하다, 채우다
to complete paperwork

form *n.* 서식
a sheet of paper

take *v.* (시간이) 걸리다
to require a certain amount of time

insurance *n.* 보험
coverage in case of a problem

complete *v.* (서식을 빠짐없이) 기입하다, 작성하다
to finish; to fill out in full

bring ~ back ~을 돌려주다
to return

be finished 끝나다
to be done

bother *v.* 괴롭히다, 신경 쓰이게 하다
to annoy; to cause pain or annoyance

come down with (가벼운 병 등에) 걸리다
to become sick

symptom *n.* 증상
a sign of an illness or sickness

sore *adj.* 아픈, 따가운
hurt; painful

throat *n.* 목구멍
the front inside part of the neck

runny *adj.* 콧물이 흐르는
dripping; releasing mucus from the nose

plugged up 꽉 막힌
stuffed up; stopped up

temperature *n.* (몸의) 고열; 체온
a fever; hotness in the body that is higher than normal

ache *n.* 아픔, 쑤심
a continuous pain that is not very strong

pulse *n.* 맥박
the number of times per minute that a person's heart beats

pop *v.* (귀가) 뚫리다
to open with a short sound

slight *adj.* 경미한, 약간의
minor; small

fever *n.* 열
a condition in which the body is hotter than normal

Unit 03

blood pressure *n.* 혈압
the pressure of the blood against the body's blood vessels

roll up ~을 걷다, 올리다
to turn up

press *v.* 누르다
to push down on

normal *adj.* 정상적인, 보통의
average; usual

step on ~에 올라서다
to put one's foot or feet onto

scale *n.* 체중계
a device that measures weight

put on weight 체중이 늘다
to get heavier; to gain weight

bowel movement *n.* 배변
the act of removing solid waste from the body

loose *adj.* 설사기가 있는, 흐물흐물한
runny

lose weight 체중이 줄다
to get lighter

watery *adj.* 묽은, 물기가 많은
liquid

belly *n.* 배
stomach

lower *adj.* 아래쪽의
below something of the same kind

mostly *adv.* 주로
usually; commonly

center *n.* 한가운데, 중심
the middle

constant *adj.* 지속적인, 끊임없는
continual; not stopping

sharp *adj.* 찌르는 듯한
painful; intense

go away 사라지다
to leave; to stop

get worse 더 나빠지다, 악화하다
to become very bad

appendicitis *n.* 맹장염
the inflammation of the appendix

Unit 04

give ~ directions ~에게 길을 가르쳐 주다
to provide instructions on how to get to a place

department *n.* 과, 부서
a section; a unit

look for ~을 찾다
to try to find; to search for

cardiology *n.* 심장학
the study of the heart

be located 있다
to be in a certain place

floor *n.* 층
a story; one level in a building

by *prep.* ~ 옆에
next to; beside

nurses' station *n.* 간호사실
an area in a hospital where many nurses stay

take *v.* (탈것에) 타다
to ride on; to use

get off ~에서 내리다
to get out of; to leave

turn left 좌회전하다
to move to one's left

hall *n.* 복도; 현관
a long passageway in a building

in front of ~ 앞에
before

give a hand 도와 주다, 거들어 주다
to help; to assist

maternity ward *n.* 산부인과 병동
a section in a hospital in which pregnant mothers and babies are taken care of

find one's way 길을 찾아가다
to get to a place by oneself

spell *v.* (어떤 단어의) 철자를 말하다
to say or write the letters in a word correctly

front door *n.* 정문
the main door of a building

get lost 길을 잃다
not to know where one is

be hospitalized 입원하다
to be in a hospital to receive medical care

Unit 05

order *v.* 지시하다
to tell a person to do something

run *v.* (테스트·검사 등을) 하다
to conduct; to do something such as a test

draw blood 피를 뽑다
to remove blood from a person's body

take a seat 앉다
to sit down

make a fist 주먹을 쥐다
to close one's hand so that it forms a fist

sting *n.* 찌르는 듯한 아픔
a sudden, sharp pain

bandage *n.* 붕대
a piece of cloth used to keep a cut or wound from bleeding

dizzy *adj.* 어지러운
spinning; unable to see straight because everything is spinning or moving

ask *v.* 요청하다, 부탁하다
to request; to question

needle *n.* (주사) 바늘
a small, sharp pointed, metal object used to pierce the skin

hold out (손 등을) 내밀다
to extend

sit back 편안히 앉다
to lie back and to relax

barely *adv.* 거의 ~않게
hardly; almost not at all

lightheaded *adj.* 약간 어지러운
faint; feeling like one is going to pass out

in no time 곧
soon

conduct *v.* 실시하다
to run; to do

urine *n.* 소변
liquid waste from the body; pee

stool *n.* 대변
solid waste from the body; feces

container *n.* 용기, 그릇
a jar, bottle, or other similar object used to keep things in

label *n.* (물건의 정보를 붙여 놓은) 라벨
a piece of paper or something similar with information on it and which is placed on a package, box, container, etc.

Unit 06

scan *n.* 정밀 검사
an exam; a test

wear *v.* 착용하다
to have on clothes or accessories

remove *v.* (옷 등을) 벗다; 제거하다
to take off

set aside ~을 한쪽으로 치워 놓다
to put something somewhere else

metallic *adj.* 금속으로 된
made of metal

lie down 눕다
to lie back on a flat surface

lie on one's back 드러눕다
to rest so that one is on one's back and looking up

remain still 가만히 있다
not to move; to keep from moving

be over 끝나다
to finish; to end

entire *adj.* 전체의
complete; total; all

ultrasound *n.* 초음파
an exam that uses sound waves to see inside the body

swelling *n.* 부기, 부어오른 곳
a part of the body that has grown larger than normal

examination table *n.* 진찰대
a table that a patient sits or lies on while a doctor exams that person

pull ~ up ~을 올리다
to lift

rub *v.* (크림 등을 문지르며) 바르다
to move one's hand back and forth on something

jelly *n.* 젤리형 크림, 젤 타입으로 된 것
a semisolid substance

produce *v.* 만들어 내다
to make

transducer *n.* (에너지) 변환기
a device that gets a signal in one type of energy and changes it to another form of energy

expose *v.* 드러내다
to show

transmit *v.* 전송하다
to send

Unit 07

bedside table *n.* 침대 옆 탁자
a small table that is located next to a bed

call button *n.* 호출 버튼
a button that makes a sound to attract a person when it is pushed

press *v.* 누르다
to push

pain medicine *n.* 진통제
a pain reliever; medication that makes a person feel less pain

serve *v.* 제공하다
to give food to

visiting hours *n.* 면회 시간
the times when people can visit a place such as a hospital

weekdays *n.* 평일
Monday through Friday

recover *v.* 회복하다
to get better

be in pain 아파하다, 고통스러워하다
to hurt; to experience pain

noon *n.* 정오, 낮 12시
twelve o'clock during the day

run *v.* (특정한 시간 동안) 계속되다
to go from one time to another

last *v.* (특정한 시간 동안) 계속되다
to go from one time to another

pillow *n.* 베개
a soft cushion one can put one's head on to sleep

provide *v.* 제공하다, 지급하다
to give to; to serve

soy milk *n.* 두유
a type of liquid made from soybeans

regular *adj.* 일반적인, 보통의
normal; usual

dietician *n.* 영양사
an expert on nutrition

toiletries *n.* 세면도구
items used in the bathroom such as soap, shampoo, and toothpaste

convenience store *n.* 편의점
a small store open 24 hours a day that sells food and practical items

basement *n.* 지하층
an underground floor in a building

Unit 08

dressing *n.* (상처 위에 덮는) 드레싱, 붕대
material used to cover a cut or a wound

itch *v.* 가렵다, 근질근질하다
to have a feeling on the skin that one wants to scratch

replace *v.* 갈다, 교체하다
to change one thing for another

sterile *adj.* 소독한, 살균한
clean; having no germs

cut *n.* (베이거나 긁힌) 상처
a wound in the skin; a part of the skin that has been opened

heal *v.* 낫다, 치유되다
to get better

infected *adj.* 감염된
having harmful germs

appear to ~인 것 같다
to seem

improve *v.* 나아지다
to get better

rapidly *adv.* 급속히, 빨리
quickly; fast; swiftly

position *n.* 자세
the way in which one is sitting or lying down

decrease *v.* 줄이다
to lower

blood flow *n.* 혈류(량)
the movement of blood in the body

tissue *n.* 조직
fleshy parts of the body

weak *adj.* 약한
not strong; having little or no strength or energy

bedsore *n.* 욕창
a sore one gets from lying in bed for too long

rotate *v.* 회전하다; 교대로 하다
to turn; to move around

turn around 몸을 돌리다
to change positions

frequently *adv.* 자주
often

in that case 그렇다면
therefore; so

Unit 09

side effect *n.* 부작용
an effect of medicine that is different from its intended effect

give ~ a shot ~에게 주사를 놓다
to put a needle into someone's body and then to inject medicine; to give an injection

IV drip *n.* 정맥 내 투여기
a tool that lets liquid enter the body through a tube and a needle

drowsy *adj.* 졸린, 졸음이 오는
sleepy; feeling like one needs to sleep

nauseous *adj.* 메스꺼운, 구역질나는
feeling like one is sick or is going to throw up

develop *v.* (병·문제가) 생기다
to get some kind of a problem

skin rash *n.* 피부 발진
a condition in which red spots appear on the skin

adjust *v.* 조절하다
to change

pill *n.* 알약
medicine taken in a solid form

blood clot *n.* 혈전
a mass or lump of blood in the body

form *v.* 형성되다, 생기다
to develop; to come into being

lower *v.* 낮추다
to decrease; to make less

pain medication *n.* 진통제
medicine that reduces the amount of pain one feels

commonly *adv.* 보통, 흔히
usually; normally

on an empty stomach 공복에
without having eaten; having no food in one's body

upset *v.* 상하게 하다
to make sick or ill

vomit *v.* 토하다, 게우다
to throw up; to expel solid or liquid matter from one's body through the mouth

organ *n.* 장기
a group of tissues in the body, such as the heart, liver, and brain, that perform an important function

transplant *n.* 이식
the operation of moving an organ from one place to another

throw up 토하다, 게우다
to vomit; to expel solid or liquid matter from one's body through the mouth

Unit 10

reassure *v.* 안심시키다
to make a person feel better

awake *adj.* 잠이 깬, 깨어 있는
not sleeping; alert

recovery room *n.* 회복실
a place in a hospital for patients after they have had surgery

groggy *adj.* 정신이 혼미한
dazed; unable to think clearly

anesthesia *n.* 마취
the use of a drug that removes feeling from the body so that a medical procedure can be performed

wear off 사라지다, 없어지다
no longer to be effective or working; to stop working

chest *n.* 가슴, 흉부
the part of the body going from the neck to the abdomen

hurt *v.* 아프다
to be in painful; to experience pain

dry *adj.* 마른, 건조한
having no moisture; not wet

operation *n.* 수술
surgery; a medical procedure in which a doctor enters a patient's body to do something

go well 잘되다
to be successful

awful *adj.* 끔찍한, 지독한
very bad

feel sore 아프다
to ache; to have pain

badly *adv.* 심하게
poorly; not well

go *v.* (일의 진행이 어떻게) 되다
to proceed; to happen

guardian *n.* 보호자; 후견인
a person who looks after another one, such as an adult who looks after a child

complication *n.* 문제
a problem

work out (일이) 잘 풀리다
to go well; to be successful

surgeon *n.* 외과 의사
a doctor who performs surgery

successful *adj.* 성공적인
winning; having been done well or properly

Unit 11

inform *v.* 알리다
to tell a person about something

dos and don'ts *n.* 주의사항
actions or activities that people should or should not do

be discharged 퇴원하다
to be sent home from the hospital

take *v.* (약을) 먹다, 복용하다
to consume medicine

cough *v.* 기침하다
to remove air from the lungs by making a harsh sound

abdomen *n.* 배, 복부
the stomach

ease *v.* (고통 등을) 덜어 주다
to make better; to make less painful

stride *n.* 보폭
a step

daily *adv.* 매일, 날마다
every day

after meals 식후에
after eating food

pay *v.* 지불하다
to give money for a good or service

bill *n.* 청구서, 계산서
a piece of paper showing how much one owes or paid

insurance card *n.* 보험증
a card showing that one has some type of insurance

information *n.* 정보
knowledge

record *n.* 기록
written information about something

cover *v.* (보험으로) 보장하다
to pay for the cost of something

cost *n.* 비용
a price; the amount of money needed to pay for a good or service

be responsible for ~에 책임이 있다
to have to take care of or do something

rest *n.* 나머지
the remainder

on file 기록되어, 보관되어
recorded; having a record of something

Unit 12

perform *v.* 행하다, 실시하다
to do; to act

medicine *n.* 약
a substance that can improve a person's condition

prescription *n.* 처방전
directions for a pharmacist to provide a person with medication

a week's worth of 1주일치의
enough for one week

make an appointment (진료) 예약을 하다
to set a time and day to do something

outpatient clinic *n.* 외래병동
a healthcare center that treats patients who do not need to be hospitalized

operate *v.* 수술하다
to do surgery

be out of ~이 다 떨어지다
not to have; to have run out of

prescribe *v.* 처방하다
to give instructions for a person to take some kind of medication

complain *v.* (고통·병 등을) 호소하다
to say that something is bothering one

treat *v.* 치료하다
to deal with a sickness, illness, or problem to make it go away or be better

minor *adj.* 작은, 가벼운
small; not important

headache *n.* 두통
a condition in which one's head hurts

fever *n.* 열
a condition in which one's body is hotter than normal

work *v.* 효과가 있다
to have an effect on

wonder *v.* 궁금해하다
to be curious about; to want to know the answer to a question

call back (전화를 해 왔던 사람에게) 다시 전화하다
to make a return telephone call

slight *adj.* 약간의, 경미한
small; minor

help *v.* 도움이 되다
to work; to be effective

visit *v.* 방문하다, 찾아가다
to go to see someone